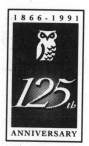

1866-1991

125th

ANNIVERSARY

D0000183

ACUPRESSURE
FOR EVERYBODY

ACUPRESSURE FOR EVERYBODY

GENTLE,

EFFECTIVE RELIEF

FOR MORE THAN

100 COMMON

AILMENTS

Cathryn Bauer

Illustrated by Jackie Aher

An Owl Book
HENRY HOLT AND COMPANY
New York

Published by Henry Holt and Company, Inc.,
115 West 18th Street, New York, New York 10011.
Published in Canada by Fitzhenry & Whiteside Limited,
195 Allstate Parkway, Markham, Ontario L3R 4T8.

Library of Congress Cataloging-in-Publication Data
Bauer, Cathryn.
Acupressure for everybody : gentle, effective relief for more
than 100 common ailments / Cathryn Bauer.—1st American ed.
p.   cm.
Includes bibliographical references and index.
ISBN 0-8050-1579-5
1. Acupressure.   I. Title.
RM723.A27B378   1991
615.8'22—dc20   90-25135
CIP

Henry Holt books are available at special discounts
for bulk purchases for sales promotions, premiums,
fund-raising, or educational use. Special editions
or book excerpts can also be created to specification.
For details contact:
Special Sales Director, Henry Holt and Company, Inc.,
115 West 18th Street, New York, New York 10011

First Edition

Designed by Katy Riegel
Printed in the United States of America
Recognizing the importance of preserving
the written word, Henry Holt and Company, Inc.,
by policy, prints all of its first editions
on acid-free paper. ∞

1   3   5   7   9   10   8   6   4   2
The author gratefully acknowledges Summit Books
for their permission to use the quotation on page 13.

This book is dedicated to Theodore Kahn.
"Many waters cannot quench love;
no flood can sweep it away."
—Song of Songs 8:7

Acknowledgments

Much gratitude is due to the following persons who believed in this book:

Dominick Abel, literary agent extraordinaire, who persevered in the face of defeat;

Theresa Burns, editor at Henry Holt and Company, Inc., who understood its message at once and helped me bring it to final form;

Crunch Software Corporation, which loaned word processing equipment and expertise;

Margot Edwards, John Gill, and Elaine Goldman Gill, who taught me so much about putting ideas on paper;

Ping Lee, who taught me Shiatsu and deepened my understanding of Asian health theory;

Janet Acuna, Hedy Babka, Donna Smith, Renee Wojnowski, Christine Kojima, and Father Isaiah Teichert for their years of encouragement and companionship.

Contents

List of Illustrations   viii
Common Ailments at a Glance   ix
Foreword
    Martin Rossman, M.D.   xiii

Introduction   1
1   Touch for Healing: The Western View
    of Acupressure   7
2   The Five Elements: The Eastern View
    of Acupressure   12
3   The Golden Points: Using Acupressure   18
4   Common Ailments A–Z   40
5   Acupressure for Infants and Children   102
6   Acupressure for People Sixty or Better   119
7   Supplements to Acupressure   124

Resources   131
References   135
Index   139

List of Illustrations

ACUPRESSURE POINTS

Acupressure Points on the Front of the Body   26
Acupressure Points on the Back of the Body   27
Acupressure Points on the Sides of the Head   28
Acupressure Points on the Face   29
Acupressure Points on the Back of the Head   30
Acupressure Points on the Hand   31
Acupressure Points on the Inside and Outside of the Foot   32
Acupressure Points on Top and Bottom of the Foot   33

GOLDEN POINTS

Golden Points on the Front of the Body   34
Golden Points on the Back of the Body   35
Golden Points on Head Region   36
Golden Points on the Hand   37
Golden Points on the Foot   38–39

Acupressure Points on an Infant   104–105
Stretching Exercises   129

Common Ailments
at a Glance

Abrasions
  (Scrapes)   40
Acne   41
Altitude Sickness   41
Anal Fissure   42
Anxiety   42
Asthma   44
Back Pain and
  Tension   44
Balanitis (Foreskin
  Inflammation)   45
Bed-wetting (Urinary
  Incontinence)   98
Bee Stings   76
Bladder Symptoms   46

Bleeding   47
Blisters   48
Boils   48
Breastfeeding
  Problems   106
Breathing Difficulties   49
Bruises   49
Bruxism (Tooth
  Grinding)   50
Burns   50
Bursitis (Joint
  Pain and Stiffness)   78
Calluses and Corns   51
Canker Sores   52
Chapped Skin   52

Chicken Pox	106	Gout	69
Claustrophobia	53	Hay Fever	69
Cold Hands and Feet	53	Headache	70
Colds and Bronchitis	54	Heartburn	71
Colic	107	Hemorrhoids	71
Conjunctivitis		Hernia	72
(Pinkeye)	56	Herpes	73
Constipation	57	Hives	73
Contact Dermatitis		Hyperventilation	113
(Rash)	58	Impetigo (Pyoderma)	114
Convulsions	108	Impotence	74
Cradle Cap	109	Influenza (Flu)	75
Cramps	58	Injection Pain	76
Croup	110	Insect Stings	76
Dehydration	111	Insomnia	77
Depression	59	Jock Rot	77
Diaper Rash (Prickly		Joint Pain and	
Heat)	112	Stiffness	78
Diarrhea	60	Knee Injury	79
Dry Eyes	61	Laryngitis	81
Ear Discomfort	61	Liver Pain	82
Eczema	62	Measles	114
Epididymitis (Scrotum		Menstrual Cramps	83
Inflammation and		Menopausal	
Infection)	63	Symptoms	121
Excessive Perspiration	63	Monilia (Yeast	
Eyestrain	64	Infection)	83
Fainting	65	Mumps	115
Fatigue	65	Nasal Congestion	84
Fever	66	Nausea	84
Flatulence	67	Nosebleed	115
Foot Pain	68	Panic	85
Foreskin Inflammation		Pelvic Pain	86
(Balanitis)	45	Penis Irritation	87

Pharyngitis (Sore Throat) 87
Pinkeye
  (Conjunctivitis)   56
Poison Exposure or
  Ingestion   88
Poison Oak, Ivy, or
  Sumac   89
Prickly Heat   112
Prostate Symptoms   90
Psoriasis   90
Pyoderma (Impetigo)   114
Rash (Contact
  Dermatitis)   58
Scrapes (Abrasions)   40
Scrotum Inflammation
  and Infection
  (Epididymitis)   63
Shin Splints   91
Shock   92
Shoulder Stiffness   78
Smoke Inhalation   93
Sore Throat
  (Pharyngitis)   87
Stitch in the Side   94

Stomach/Abdominal
  Discomfort   94
Stress   95
Teething   116
Tennis Elbow
  (Tendonitis)   96
Testicle Torsion   97
Tonsillitis   117
Toothache   97
Tooth Grinding
  (Bruxism)   50
Umbilical Cord
  Infection   117
Urinary Incontinence
  (Bed-wetting)   98
Vaginal Discharge and
  Itching   118
Varicose Veins   98
Vertigo   99
Vomiting   100
Whiplash   100
Yeast Infection
  (Monilia)   83

Foreword

In 1971 I saw a videotape that dramatically changed the way I practiced medicine. The videotape was made in China by a blue-ribbon delegation of medical scientists from the American Medical Association. It showed a young man having part of his lung removed while fully conscious, with only several small acupuncture needles being used for anesthesia. While the surgeon cut through the patient's ribs, a nurse was feeding him sections of mandarin oranges and sips of tea. At the end of the operation, the man was bandaged, sat up, and walked out of the operating room.

The AMA delegation witnessed many such operations and concluded that while they didn't understand what was going on, the phenomenon of acupuncture was real and "deserved serious investigation" by the Western scientific community. While some acupuncture research has since been performed in the West, the great bulk of it has been carried out in Europe and China. During this time, we have learned that acupuncture stimulates the release of endorphins—which are not only natural painkillers but also mood and immune system regulators—as well as a host of other neurohormones and chemical transmitters that have profound effects on the body and mind. Today, acupuncture is not only alive and well in the Orient, it is a growing, thriving health profession in Europe and the United States. There is an American Medical Acupuncture Association, and a National Commission for the Certification of Acupuncturists has established criteria for national board certification. Millions of Westerners have been successfully treated with acupuncture for problems as diverse as chronic pain, allergies, arthritis, asthma, menstrual difficulties, anxiety, and depression.

While acupuncture should be administered by health professionals with years of training and experience, *acupressure,* which utilizes the same system of stimulating certain points on the body to activate healing responses, is a wonderful self-care tool. In the Orient, acupressure and Shiatsu (a Japanese variant of acupressure) are widely used for relaxation, health maintenance, and self-treatment of many common illnesses and symptoms. It might be thought of as the equivalent of our "over-the-counter" medicines.

In this clear, straightforward book, Cathryn Bauer has given us the instruction we need in order to put this marvelous healing tool to good use. With plain language—and useful illustrations—she makes acupressure treatment available to anyone willing to invest a small amount of time and sensitivity to working with themselves or their loved ones. She offers prescriptions for treating many common causes of suffering and has even included special sections for working with children, the elderly, and the disabled. Admirably, she has also taken care to point out safety precautions when working with acupressure, mostly having to do with not using it inappropriately as a replacement for good medical care.

This is an extremely helpful book that I will recommend to many of my patients. Take the time to experiment with what Cathryn Bauer has offered here, and I'm sure you will be rewarded with an increased sense of well-being, vitality, and good health, as well as an increased sense of confidence and awe for the remarkable self-healing abilities of your body.

Martin L. Rossman, M.D.
Mill Valley, California, April 1991

Introduction

Two years ago I took part in a rafting expedition on the Lower Klamath River in Northern California with eleven other adults. On the last day of the trip, one of our guides was stung by a wasp while she prepared lunch. I had thought the appropriate remedy for insect bites was common knowledge. But when I saw her simply putting her finger to her mouth while she continued making sandwiches with her other hand, all the while groaning with pain, I thought I'd better act. I told her to rinse the injury while I crushed some ice cubes on a rock. Then I fastened the ice over the sting with a cloth napkin.

"Keep it there ten minutes," I instructed, "so it won't swell. It'll stop hurting very soon." Another guide took over lunch preparations. I massaged the base of the stung finger to stimulate circulation, then pressed the acupressure points Heart 7 and Pericardium 8 for shock. Ten minutes later, she held up her hand in amazement. "No swelling, and it feels like it never happened. How did you do that?"

This incident made me realize how few people know of the

wealth of natural remedies available for common ailments. One of the most powerful and effective of these is acupressure. This ancient health art, which originated in China thousands of years ago, can provide fast symptom relief in numerous situations of physical, as well as psychological, discomfort. It requires no special tools aside from knowledge, sensitivity, and concentration, which makes it a useful and accessible resource for travelers, people with drug allergies, pregnant and lactating women, and just about everyone else.

I originally became interested in acupressure about ten years ago, because its philosophy—the Five Elements Theory—seemed a fine blueprint for healthy living. (I discuss this philosophy in Chapter 2.) I felt that its guidelines for adapting life-styles to the seasons could help prevent disease of body and emotions. I was also very impressed with acupressure's effectiveness in pain and tension relief. I once received a massage while recovering from a migraine headache. The masseuse, an acupressure student, gently pressed and held a point inside my ankle (Kidney 3). My residual pain faded dramatically, and did not return. I felt warmer and stronger. After the massage, I went home and slept deeply for ten hours. I woke the next morning with only a fraction of my usual post-migraine weakness and irritability.

I wanted to learn more about this remarkable treatment, so I enrolled in a bodywork course to study touch therapy in its various forms: pressing acupressure points, Shiatsu (a vigorous massage involving pressing, squeezing, and kneading of tight muscles), and Swedish/Esalen massage, which involved stroking warm oil into the muscles.

Acupressure was an exciting discovery. Yet I observed some disturbing trends within the "holistic" community during my certification work, including a rejection of conventional medical knowledge and a "blame the victim" mentality. It seemed that I was being trained to work with one composite client: a youthful adult without serious medical problems or reservations about alternative health and bodywork therapies. There was no discussion of medical conditions that might require me to modify the recommended treatment patterns. In addition, students were not well supervised while pressing points in class. Another Shiatsu student forced my hip joint after I told her, "That's enough. Don't press back anymore." The injury that followed was painful, although short term. My complaint to the instructor was ignored, and she was never counseled about her failure to respond to me.

After I completed the requirements for certification, I began to study paramedic and nursing textbooks on my own. I pored over a skeleton model, anatomy charts, and acupuncture diagrams. I searched unsuccessfully for material on the Five Elements Theory, and how its unique concepts could be applied to the lives of Westerners, then decided to pursue methods its originators might have used. These included daily reflection on each of the elements and its role in nature, particularly human nature. I also kept notebooks to record their manifestations in my clients and myself, and studied other natural healing techniques, including herbalism.

This study led to a successful private practice in the San Francisco Bay area. Clients brought a wide variety of physical and emotional ailments to my treatment table. In any given week, among other ailments I might see severe menstrual discomfort, arthritis pain, and post-surgical fatigue. Some clients chose to receive regular bodywork for stress reduction. A young restaurant owner received weekly sessions to counteract the effects of his seven days a week career. A law student routinely called me at exam time.

I also learned the value of self-treatment during the early years of my practice. In 1982 my car was struck from behind. The accident left me with a neuroma, or chronic pain and sensitivity, on the inside of one calf and I limped, a condition my orthopedist told me I'd be "stuck with." Acupressure formed the cornerstone of an aggressive self-care program that included visualization, herbal compresses, and Tai Chi Chu'an (a yogalike Chinese exercise routine that promotes balance and relaxation). The pain and stiffness decreased sharply within seven days and disappeared completely six months later.

This experience left me with great confidence in the healing powers of acupressure. But I also encountered situations with clients that made me reflect on my *limits* as a practitioner. One man came to me following a blow to his lower back. He could not stand upright and was obviously suffering from intense pain. I was reluctant to apply finger pressure under these circumstances, and asked him to get X rays before we worked together. The results revealed a vertebral fracture, which showed me how conventional medical technology could sometimes give me the answers I needed to press points safely and effectively.

It was crucial for me, as an acupressurist, to recognize health problems that required a doctor's care, since clients often relied on my guidance. A Japanese-American woman sought treatment for menopausal symptoms. Tomiko's urinary incontinence made a full night's sleep impossible. This weakened her, and she was susceptible to colds and other infections. Acupressure and herbal remedies brought relief. Tomiko made it clear that she trusted me completely. She followed my instructions for between-session care to the letter and never questioned any aspect of our work. This was flattering, but I felt a sobering responsibility.

Meanwhile, many other women came to me for similar problems, and acupressure repeatedly proved itself to be particularly effective in gynecological treatment. I gave acupressure sessions to women with severe premenstrual syndrome and period pain, with good results. Robin, a single mother, was so dizzy and weak one day that I had to make an acupressure "house call." Her six-year-old son Ben answered the door and explained how glad he was to see me, since "Mom feels so bad she can't walk downstairs." Robin was suffering from violent nausea and abdominal cramps, as well as dizziness. I had her remain on the bed, and the three of us went to work. Ben stroked his mother's hand while I pressed Spleen 10 for fifteen minutes. We concentrated on imagining Robin feeling all well and able to go outside with him. It worked. Robin relaxed as the cramping pain subsided, and color returned to her face. I pressed other points for nausea and stress while Ben played quietly. When we finished, he escorted me to the door and said, "Thank you for helping my mom!"

I was glad to help Ben's mom, but what I really wanted was to help my female clients take care of themselves when I was unavailable. I had also discovered that sessions were most empowering for all clients when they included self-care instruction. So I began to teach classes, giving out charts and instruction sheets as a sort of homework. With feedback from my students, these charts and instruction sheets expanded, eventually forming the basis of my first book, *Acupressure for Women*.

The response from women who read my book was gratifying. Yet more and more men were expressing an interest in acupressure, and asked for material that addressed their particular needs. (My cousin Eddie said, "I loved it. Now write one for me.") I began to think about an acupressure text that was appropriate for all of my other clients, which included not only men, but young children and the elderly as well.

In *Acupressure for Everybody*, I've tried to place the healing powers of this technique into the hands of the greatest number of people, regardless of sex or age or state of health. It includes instructions for the relief of over 100 common ailments, as well as advice on emotional care for the injured and ill. While it cannot promise miracles, acupressure can provide a gentle first-aid kit at your fingertips. This book will show you how it can be practiced safely and with care.

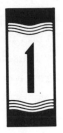

Touch for Healing:
The Western View of Acupressure

For the last several decades, Western society has been developing a new understanding of the causes and treatments in physical and emotional disease. We now challenge the traditional emphasis placed on technology, and increasingly perceive the medical model of symptom-focused treatment as incomplete. This, in turn, has led to a greater interest in therapies that positively affect our emotional states. Relaxation techniques such as acupressure, fundamental in Asian health care, are gaining an appreciative Western audience. Many clients have come to me for acupressure treatment with a goal such as "getting to the real cause of this fatigue/shoulder tension/problem with my wrist." Others seek help with symptoms such as chronic digestive discomfort, insomnia, and anxiety.

Acupressure is a relaxing natural therapy that teaches the body to identify and release patterns of holding tension. An established body of evidence supports its effectiveness in symptom relief and stress reduction.

In the 1950s, Hans Selye, M.D., showed that emotional states affect health. A fearful response to stressful situations puts us into "fight or flight syndrome," where we see either battle or escape as our sole alternative. Our bodies respond accordingly, preparing for self-defense or escape with elevated blood pressure, pounding heart, and tense, action-ready muscles. We remain in this state until the perceived threat is resolved. Fight or flight syndrome can last for seconds, days, or years. Dr. Selye associated chronic stress of this nature with illnesses like gastric ulcer, hypertension, and migraine, and encouraged patients to adopt alternatives to the fight or flight stance.

Dr. Selye's findings inspired other medical researchers to study relaxation techniques such as biofeedback, hypnosis, and mental imaging. At Harvard University, Herbert Benson, M.D., adapted Eastern meditation practices into a stress-release program he called the relaxation response. Studies proved that hypertensives who practiced his technique while consuming a low-cholesterol, fiber-rich diet could sharply reduce their blood pressure with little or no prescribed medication. Dean Ornish, M.D., author of *Stress, Diet and Your Heart*, carried Dr. Benson's ideas further. He found that relaxation training lessened the severity of angina attacks and lowered bloodstream cholesterol levels. Duke University researchers studied the effects of biofeedback training on diabetic patients. They found that subjects who learned to relax their muscles at will also showed an increased ability to regulate their blood sugar levels.

We instinctively touch when we want to comfort and heal. Shiatsu, a vigorous style of massage, is a routine part of wellness maintenance for many Asian families. India's Ayurvedic medical practitioners rub herbs and oils into their patients' skins. Massage, the touch therapy best known to Westerners, is increasingly used to alleviate stress symptoms such as muscular tension. Sugar Ray Leonard received daily massage and acupressure treatments while training for the World Middleweight Boxing Championship in 1987. His masseur also coached him in deep-breathing techniques. Leonard's trainer felt this relaxed his muscles and helped him to break the stamina-draining habit of holding his breath during a fight.

Relaxing touch therapies have also found their way into hospital care. A few nurse-midwives regularly use acupressure to ease pain, fatigue, and tension during labor. A growing number of nurses have adopted a technique called Therapeutic Touch, developed by Dolores Krieger, R.N. Krieger-trained practitioners place their hands on or near the body of the patient and move them in long, stroking motions. Krieger claims this renews and balances the energy field surrounding the body. Studies verify that Therapeutic Touch helps patients to relax and helps to improve psychophysical recovery. A control group of hospitalized patients who received Therapeutic Touch as part of routine nursing care demonstrated a significant increase in blood hemoglobin (iron) levels, indicating increased stamina and healing capacity. Another patient group was given standardized self-assessment questionnaires to determine their anxiety levels prior to a Therapeutic Touch session. The questionnaires were given again after the session, and the results showed a marked drop in patient anxiety.

There are several reasons why touch therapies promote calmness and clarity. Since a tense muscle is more painful than one that is relaxed and flexible, a trained touch may have direct physiological benefits. Touch therapies such as massage and acupressure relieve muscle tension, eliminating problems like inhibited circulation. Research also suggests that touch therapies benefit the nervous system.

Some neurologists believe the skin surface contains sensitive neural receptors, also theorized as acupressure points. David Bresler, M.D., director of the Pain Control Unit at the University of California, Los Angeles, says that pressing these neural receptors affects heart rate, blood flow, and endocrine function. Dr. Bruce Pomeranz of the University of Toronto found that stimulating the neural receptors prompts the brain to release its own painkilling hormones, endorphins, which are structurally similar to morphine. Neural receptor stimulation probably works in much the same way. Researchers speculate further that painkilling drugs activate the brain's analgesic mechanisms, the inhibitory and excitatory pleasure centers. Your inhibitory center enables you to relax and feel secure. When it is activated, you rest comfortably and avoid fatigue and tension buildup. The excitatory pleasure center stimulates self-confidence and your ability to take charge of a situation.

You can use acupressure to stimulate neural receptor sites. Acupressure is convenient for minor emergencies, too, as it requires no special tools other than knowledge and concentration to promote relaxation and ease uncomfortable symptoms. For example, David, a client, used acupressure while backpacking to ease his nausea and dizziness in recovering from a bout with altitude sickness.

Acupressure treatments consist of slow, gradual finger pressure applied to neural receptor sites. (These are the same points an acupuncturist treats with needles.) Asian medical practitioners believe that the points are located on meridian paths that distribute life energy throughout your body. Disease, or dis-ease, symptoms of body, mind, and spirit occur when energy is blocked or otherwise imbalanced.

Acupressure points are used to balance the meridians and, thus, relieve symptoms. For maximum benefit, it is sometimes supplemented by other touch therapies and natural treatments such as herbalism (see Chapter 7, "Supplements to Acupressure").

My own therapeutic work combines acupressure with massage, a deeply relaxing technique that stimulates circulation. Massage receivers lie on a table, carpet, or bed while their muscles are stroked with warm oil. I found that clients who had recently experienced trauma (such as a car accident or surgery) relaxed more quickly when I began their session with massage. With clients who have difficulty settling into a session, I often use Shiatsu. In this form of acupressure, receivers lie on a futon (a

Japanese floor mat) while their muscles are pressed, squeezed, and kneaded. Joint tension is relieved by rotating and pulling the arms and legs. (Shiatsu is an intense form of massage that is unsuitable for clients who are ill, weak, or pregnant.)

Acupressure is sometimes used to support conventional medical treatment. Norman, a paramedic with some knowledge of acupressure, regularly presses points on trauma patients to help prevent shock. Lisa had a friend give her an acupressure session the day after her surgery. She reported, "It seemed like the clouds from the anesthesia went away. I had better control over what was happening after that."

Acupressure adds a new dimension to regular medical care, *though it cannot replace it.* You can learn to use acupressure for relaxation, improved circulation, and pain and tension control. For maximum benefit, develop an understanding of the Eastern view of acupressure described in Chapter 2, and memorize the often-used Golden Points in Chapter 3.

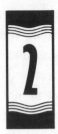

The Five Elements:
The Eastern View of Acupressure

Acupressure began in ancient China with the observation that we instinctively touch injuries. Pressing and rubbing a painful area usually provides a little relief. Sages and physicians conducted detailed studies of finger pressure's effects and discovered that pressing specific points consistently brought relief for certain conditions. In many cases, effective acupressure points were not located on, or even near, the affected body part. And so they concluded that acupressure points were connected to the various body organs they influenced. Eventually they found that the points were located on pathways of energy called *chi* that flowed through the body via predictable routes. These chi routes are known as *meridians*. This was substantiated in the early 1980s when Dr. Kim Bong-han, a Korean medical professor, showed that variations in the skin's electrical resistance could be traced along the meridians as illustrated in ancient texts. Further studies by Dr. Bong-han showed that skin cells located along the meridians were structurally unique; clusters of these meridian cells were located at the marked acupressure points.

Chi moves through our bodies via twelve major meridians. These act like rivers, carrying energy throughout the body as rivers spread water through the countryside. We also have a set of extra meridians, similar to tributaries, whose function is to receive and store excess energy for future use. The energy in the meridians constantly waxes and wanes, influenced by weather, emotion, diet, and other factors, since anything that affects health influences chi. Physical and emotional problems result from a deficiency or excess in one or more meridians. Pressing acupressure points corrects energy imbalances among the meridians, thus relieving symptoms. When chi is evenly distributed among the meridians, we are strong and resist disease.

Early researchers linked this knowledge to Taoism, a set of teachings that emphasizes unity. According to the Tao, human beings, the sun and stars, plants and animals are one entity, one fabric. All are subject to natural law. Humans reflect the physical universe, sharing in its dual aspects of earth (yin) and sky (yang).

Yin is associated with night, cold, and quiet, giving us capacities for solitude, reflection, and rest. Yang, connected with daytime, heat, and assertive action, stimulates us to physical movement and social interaction. We are yin and yang in our thinking, physical activity, and emotional processes.

We further reflect the universe in our psychophysical responses to the changing seasons. We alter physically and emotionally as the climate changes. Western research supports this ancient truism. A University of Pennsylvania study confirmed the traditional Asian view of winter as the season of withdrawal,

---

I would emphasize that Chinese . . . medicine is as logical as scientific medicine; each examines a different facet of the same person and an attempt to deal directly with his suffering.

—*Ted Kaptchuk,* The Healing Arts

---

quiet, and rest. Subjects reported that their ambition and activity levels were lowest during the winter months, with more hours of sleep. (The most severe manifestation of this has recently been labeled Seasonal Affective Disorder. SAD sufferers often need ten hours or more of sleep each night in winter.) Chinese medicine teaches that each season has other distinctive characteristics. We promote well-being by following the unique patterns of food, rest, and activity each season requires.

Each season is associated with one yin and one yang meridian, except for summer, which has two yin and two yang meridians. There are five meridian groups since the Chinese considered late summer a separate season. Each is connected to an element, one of the five essential substances forming the universe. Within ourselves they correspond to an organ, an emotion, and various other human capacities. When a meridian is imbalanced, we are most likely to experience the disease associated with its corresponding element.

We can learn to recognize the signs of each element within ourselves and identify imbalance. Then we can press acupressure points to restore a strong, steady energy flow and a state of well-being.

THE FIVE ELEMENTS

Earth

The Earth element is associated with late summer, a brief season marked by land and weather changes. Earth is the element that regulates balance, perspective, and our physical and emotional cycles. It coordinates with the Water element to create our sexuality and fertility.

The Stomach is the yang Earth meridian, governing the digestive system. The yin Earth meridian is the blood-building Spleen. A healthy Earth element regulates our physical and emotional cycles. Symptoms of imbalance include Premenstrual Syndrome, sexual dysfunction, and digestive discomfort. Earth also gives us the ability to feel sympathy. When it is balanced, we are compassionate without excusing inappropriate behavior in self or others.

Metal

Metal is the element of autumn, the harvest season, when plants give us their fruits and leaves fall. Our Metal aspect gives us the ability to acquire what we need and eliminate what is unnecessary. It stimulates us to take care of our material and spiritual needs.

The Large Intestine (yang) and the Lung (yin) are the Metal meridians. These meridians let us release what is no longer needed so that it can be replaced. When Metal is dysfunctional, you may suffer elimination problems or difficulties in breathing. Emotionally you are likely to struggle long and hard to resolve problems and difficult feelings. The Metal meridians enable us to grieve. When they are balanced, we respond appropriately to loss. We experience our grief fully, express it, and move onward.

Water

Water is the winter season. This is a time when the earth is fallow. Some animals spend the winter in hibernation. Water enables us to rest and relax in preparation for later activity. The Water meridians store energy reserves for use in future times of stress.

These reserves are held by the yin Water meridian, the Kidney. Its yang partner, the Bladder meridian, is the channel in times of physical and spiritual challenge. Water stores our reproductive energy, which permits us to have children. The Water meridians also regulate bodily fluids, bone health, hearing, and memory. Fear is the Water emotion. When it is balanced, you correctly assess threatening situations and protect yourself accordingly.

Wood

The Wood element is associated with spring, the season of new life and creativity. Wood lets us think, plan, and visualize. It is strongly associated with eye health, as well as the inner vision that helps us to design projects and bring them through to completion.

The Gall Bladder is the yang Wood meridian. It secretes bile and distributes energy from food throughout the meridian system. The Liver is the yin Wood meridian. Blood is filtered through the liver, where it is purified. This meridian also assimilates food, sorting the nutritive aspects from the nonnutritive and discarding the latter.

Anger is the Wood emotion. When Gall Bladder and Liver are strong and balanced, your anger stimulates you to constructive action, then releases harmlessly.

Fire

Summer is the season of Fire, the element that gives us an appreciation for living, is associated with our heart's well-being, and brings self-esteem. The yin Fire meridians are the Heart and its protector and nourisher, the Pericardium. The yang Fire meridians are the Small Intestine and Triple Warmer. The Small Intestine processes food, discarding wastes and distributing nutrients for maximum benefit. The Triple Warmer is the only meridian without a corresponding organ; it is an energy presence without a physical form. The Triple Warmer protects the vital centers that Chinese physicians call "the three burning spaces": the chest cavity, which includes the heart and lungs, the stomach, and the intestines. It regulates the amount of heat and nutrients these organs receive.

Fire regulates your blood circulation. If you are continually cold, your Fire meridians are probably deficient in energy. Physical diseases associated with Fire include hypertension, coronary artery disease, and angina; poor circulation, blood disorders, and difficulty with temperature changes. Emotional symptoms include depression, isolation, insensitivity to others, and low self-esteem.

Joy is the Fire emotion. When Fire is healthy, you enjoy a good laugh.

THE CONCEPTION VESSEL AND THE GOVERNING VESSEL

The Conception Vessel and the Governing Vessel are extra meridians that act as reservoirs for excess energy. Pressing points on the extra meridians helps increase the effects of an acupressure treatment. If you have excess energy and find it difficult to relax, press one or more Conception Vessel points during a treatment. Press Governing Vessel points when you feel tired or weak.

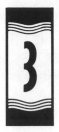

The Golden Points:
Using Acupressure

You can learn to press acupressure points to renew your energy and manage health problems. First, however, you must follow several precautions, and know how to press points sensitively.

PRECAUTIONS

Use a particularly gentle touch if you are ill, tired, or weak; abrupt application is startling, detracting from acupressure's relaxing effects.

Acupressure should never be applied directly to wounds, bruises, or sprains, since strong finger pressure may increase pain and tissue damage. However, you can press points near an injury to increase circulation and release muscular tension. Refer to the list of Golden Points to find one nearest the site of injury.

Some acupressure points should not be used during pregnancy, as they are associated with prenatal problems. They are listed on page 20, and are noted throughout the text.

HOW TO PRESS ACUPRESSURE POINTS

Your hands must be clean, warm, and dry.

Start an acupressure session by holding your palm over the

point for a moment. Then move the tip of your index finger to the point location. Probe gently until you feel a slight dip; this is the acupressure point.

Press in lightly, holding your finger in this position until you feel the muscles relax. Increase the pressure very slowly. Stop pressing when you feel that you're forcing it; just hold the pressure steady. Pay close attention to the way the point feels. Acupressure points often become warm to the touch as muscular tension eases.

Keep the pressure steady until the point is neither warm nor cool in temperature, and pulses steadily. (The pulsation is not as strong as the pulse in your wrists and neck.) This usually takes at least three minutes, and it may take ten minutes. If your symptoms are acute, the point could require even more time to release tension.

When the pulse is throbbing evenly, ease your fingertip off the point. An abrupt release of pressure feels very unpleasant to the acupressure receiver.

Some points are difficult to press on yourself. You can use an old soft tennis ball to reach points on your back. Place the ball on a carpet, and ease onto it slowly while you support yourself on your elbows.

TOUCH WITH AWARENESS

- *Ask permission before you press a point.*
- *Ask the acupressure receiver if she has injuries or some disease. Find out if she has any tender areas such as a newly healed fracture or sprain and don't work there.*
- *Let the receiver know she can ask questions about your work—and stop you if the treatment feels wrong.*
- *Make sure your hands are clean, warm, and dry.*
- *Move into the receiver's physical space slowly; an abrupt move feels threatening.*

Using acupressure is easier if you know some points' locations and uses by heart. Learn several of the points that you are most likely to use. If you have a chronic health problem such as stress headaches or asthma, you can turn to Chapter 4 and locate points and instruction written for you. If your interest in acupressure is more general (you simply like the idea of having a health kit at your fingertips), start by memorizing the Golden Points.

Ancient health scientists devised the term *Golden Points* to describe the points they used and taught most frequently. I have borrowed this phrase for points pressed to relieve common symptoms such as colds and shoulder tension. It's helpful to know by heart how to press these points, since you may need them when you are not carrying this book.

You will help others more effectively if you learn from the experience of self-care, so begin by pressing the Golden Points on yourself. Traditional Chinese acupuncture schools require stu-

---

ACUPRESSURE POINTS TO AVOID IN PREGNANCY

Do not use these points if you are pregnant, since their use is connected with prenatal difficulties such as excessive bleeding and labor pain.

Spleen 1	Stomach 4
Spleen 2	Stomach 36
Spleen 6	Stomach 45
Large Intestine 2	Lung 7
Large Intestine 4	Lung 11
Large Intestine 10	Small Intestine 7
Small Intestine 10	Kidney 1
Triple Warmer 4	Kidney 2
Triple Warmer 10	Kidney 4
Gall Bladder 2	Kidney 7
Gall Bladder 9	Pericardium 6
Pericardium 8	

---

dents to insert treatment needles into their own skin 1,000 times before they give acupuncture to patients. This is a good rule for acupressure students as well.

You should remember that symptom relief may not occur for up to thirty minutes. When you press a point, you're doing more than pressing a button. You're encouraging the large and complex meridian system to rebalance and stimulate the body's healing resources. This process takes time.

AFTER YOU PRESS POINTS

If your point location was accurate, and you applied pressure until you felt a steady pulsation, you can expect to feel more relaxed. Your breathing will be deeper. Other responses vary according to your current condition.

For example, you may want to sleep after you receive acupressure, especially if you are ill. Leslie sought acupressure treatment during a tiresome bout of gastroenteritis. She seemed restless and cranky when she appeared for her session. I pressed Small Intestine 11 for the first ten minutes. This relaxed her shoulders and chest, in addition to facilitating healthy digestion. Her stomach gurgled as I eased my fingertips off the points, and she told me, "I can feel things moving, but my stomach doesn't feel bad. It's as if it's doing what it has to do before it gets better." I moved on to Stomach 42. I pressed for five minutes before she had to get up to go to the bathroom. When she got back, I pressed points to relax her neck and shoulders, and completed the session by massaging her hands and feet. A few days later, Leslie told me, "I fell asleep as soon as I got home, and ended up sleeping for twelve hours. When I woke up, my stomach felt fine."

Other responses are also possible. If you felt restless before you pressed points, you will feel calmer and better able to focus your attention on work or recreation. (Stomach 42 and Lung 1 are particularly helpful with lack of concentration.) Repressed emotions and buried memories can sometimes surface during acupressure treatment as well. You may find yourself wanting to laugh, cry, or talk. Relax and let it happen—it's all part of the treatment.

If you're pressing points on someone else and he does begin to talk freely, be sure he knows you can be trusted to keep his confidence.

GIVING LENGTHY ACUPRESSURE TREATMENTS

You can give a brief acupressure session almost anywhere. For example, I used to give myself neck-and-shoulder treatments while riding a commuter bus. This is fine for short treatments or emergency situations. However, sometimes you want more than a quick-fix solution, particularly if you or your receiver is tired, tense, or ill. You can combine several of the treatments suggested in this book to provide a restful, nurturing experience.

Choose a time when you are unlikely to be distracted or interrupted, and dress in loose clothing. The room you work in should be quiet and warm. Find a comfortable place to lie down (you don't need an expensive massage table). You can use a sofa, lawn, padded carpet, or a firm mattress. Give your lower back some extra support by placing a pillow under your knees, and prop up your head or feet if this makes you more comfortable.

Allow your eyes to close, and take a few deep breaths. You can help to focus your attention on the session by counting backward from ten. Breathe in—let yourself see the two digits in your mind's eye. (How tall are they? What color?) Release your breath, and continue counting. When you reach zero, stop and think for a moment about what you would like to receive from this quiet time. (I always try to name three specific goals before proceeding with the session; for example, "I'd like this dull aching in my jaw to go away, I'd like to work on releasing my habit of holding tension across my scalp, and I'd like to relax my breathing.")

Then open your eyes and refer to Chapter 4. For a deeply relaxing session, you can start by pressing the points mentioned in the entries for Anxiety, page 42, Insomnia, page 77, Joint Pain and Stiffness, page 78, or Stress, page 95. Each of these point sequences is an excellent tension-reliever. If you have a specific health concern, continue by choosing points from the appropriate section in Chapter 4.

You can stop the treatment there, or you can complete it by repeating the opening sequence that you chose for general relaxation.

When you are finished pressing points, take at least a few minutes to relax completely.

THE GOLDEN POINTS

The twenty Golden Points are used for common injuries and illnesses. Practice these points until you can locate them easily, without looking at a chart. The Golden Points are used for specific health problems, as noted. You can also press the Golden Points around a wound or bruise to release muscular tension and stimulate circulation.

THE GOLDEN POINTS

Large Intestine 4 (Do not use in pregnancy): constipation, emotional release, headache.

Bladder 2: sinus congestion and headache, eye discharge, frontal headache, facial tension.

Lung 1: chest congestion, bronchitis, emotional release, stress reduction.

Stomach 42: stomach and abdominal cramps, pain from overeating, dizziness, vertigo, emotional overexcitement.

Kidney 1 (Do not use in pregnancy): fatigue, fainting, foot cramps.

Kidney 3: fatigue (especially following illness), poor stamina, low resistance to disease, ankle pain, and tension.

Gall Bladder 40: leg, foot and ankle stiffness and pain, frequent and excessive anger, indecision.

Bladder 38: shallow breathing, upper body tension, back pain and tension, emotional overexcitement.

Stomach 3: facial pain and tension, sinus congestion, toothache.

Bladder 60: sprains, foot and ankle pain, tics.

Spleen 7: itching, thigh stiffness and pain, knee injuries.

Stomach 25: diarrhea, acid indigestion, stomach cramps.

Heart 7: emotional overexcitement, depression, mood swings.

Triple Warmer 5: flu, colds, wrist and forearm pain.

Bladder 54: leg cramps, knee pain, poor circulation, varicose veins, tension and pain in the back of the legs.

Spleen 12: period pain, indigestion, hip and thigh stiffness and pain.

Bladder 42: back pain and tension, shoulder stiffness.

Gall Bladder 30: hip pain and tension, leg pain, poor leg circulation, pain from varicose veins.

Governing Vessel 16: mental clarity, headache, scalp tension.

Conception Vessel 17: emotional upset, chest constriction and congestion, upper body tension.

IN AN EMERGENCY

- *Call for emergency help immediately rather than attempt medical care you're not trained or licensed to provide.*
- *Stay calm. Remember that few injuries require instantaneous medical attention.*
- *Move the injured or ill person only if essential; for example, to get him away from a burning automobile or to remove obstacles to breathing. Otherwise, keep him as still as possible until paramedics arrive.*
- *Arrest bleeding by applying a clean cloth directly to the wound and pressing down on it with your palm until the bleeding stops.* Do not improvise a tourniquet.

- *Keep bystanders as calm as possible. Discourage unnecessary comments.*
- *Don't tell the injured person that he'll be all right (you don't know that!). Instead, reassure him that you are there to help.*
- *Encourage him to relax quietly, conserve his energy, and save his story for the authorities.*

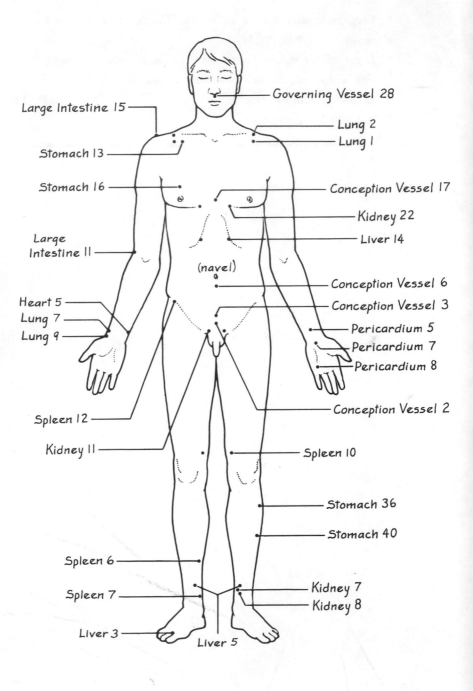

Governing Vessel 28
Large Intestine 15
Lung 2
Lung 1
Stomach 13
Stomach 16
Conception Vessel 17
Kidney 22
Liver 14
Large Intestine 11
(navel)
Conception Vessel 6
Heart 5
Conception Vessel 3
Lung 7
Lung 9
Pericardium 5
Pericardium 7
Pericardium 8
Conception Vessel 2
Spleen 12
Kidney 11
Spleen 10
Stomach 36
Stomach 40
Spleen 6
Spleen 7
Kidney 7
Kidney 8
Liver 3
Liver 5

**Acupressure Points
on the Front of the Body**

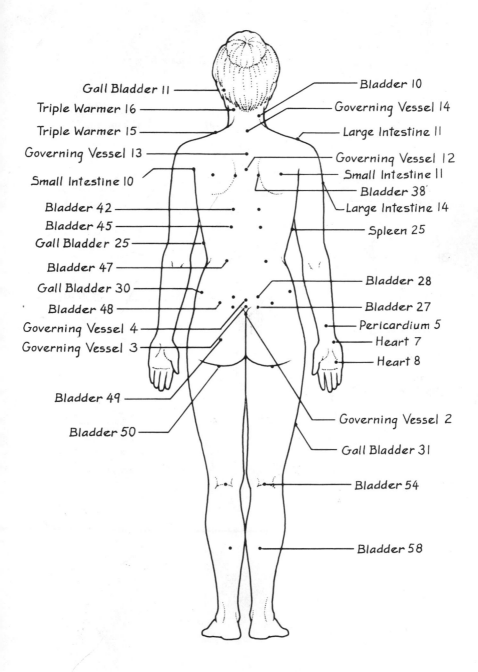

Gall Bladder 11
Triple Warmer 16
Triple Warmer 15
Governing Vessel 13
Small Intestine 10
Bladder 42
Bladder 45
Gall Bladder 25
Bladder 47
Gall Bladder 30
Bladder 48
Governing Vessel 4
Governing Vessel 3
Bladder 49
Bladder 50

Bladder 10
Governing Vessel 14
Large Intestine 11
Governing Vessel 12
Small Intestine 11
Bladder 38
Large Intestine 14
Spleen 25
Bladder 28
Bladder 27
Pericardium 5
Heart 7
Heart 8
Governing Vessel 2
Gall Bladder 31
Bladder 54
Bladder 58

**Acupressure Points
on the Back of the Body**

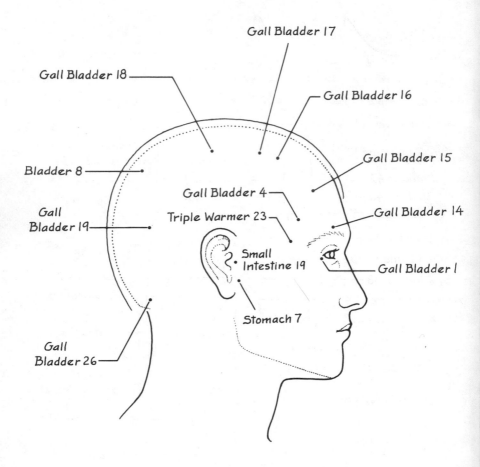

**Acupressure Points
on the Sides of the Head**

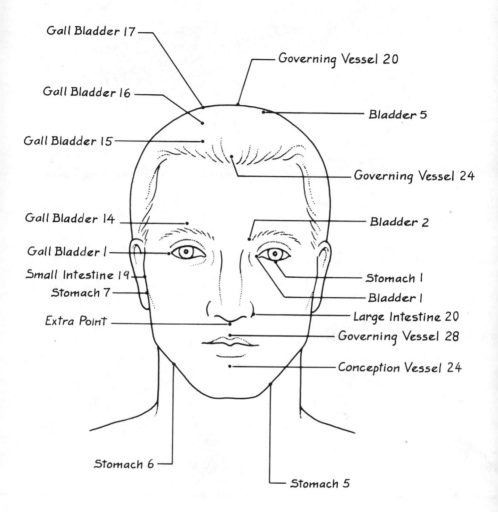

Gall Bladder 17
Gall Bladder 16
Gall Bladder 15
Gall Bladder 14
Gall Bladder 1
Small Intestine 19
Stomach 7
Extra Point
Stomach 6

Governing Vessel 20
Bladder 5
Governing Vessel 24
Bladder 2
Stomach 1
Bladder 1
Large Intestine 20
Governing Vessel 28
Conception Vessel 24
Stomach 5

**Acupressure Points
on the Face**

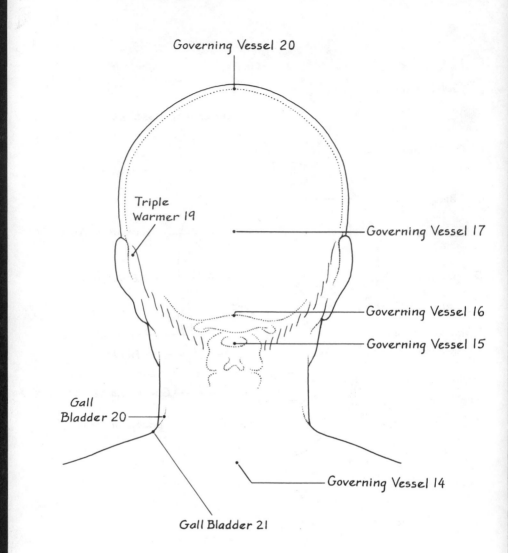

Governing Vessel 20

Triple
Warmer 19

Governing Vessel 17

Governing Vessel 16

Governing Vessel 15

Gall
Bladder 20

Governing Vessel 14

Gall Bladder 21

**Acupressure Points
on the Back of the Head**

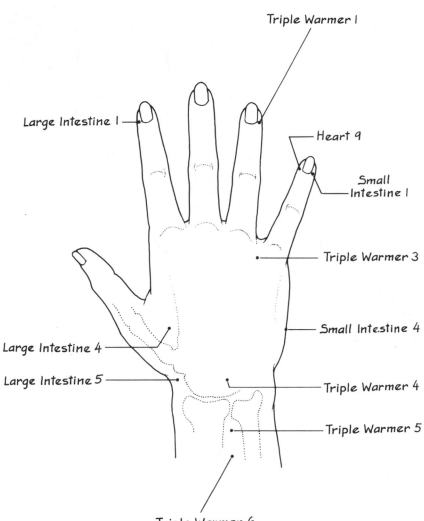

Triple Warmer 1

Large Intestine 1

Heart 9

Small
Intestine 1

Triple Warmer 3

Small Intestine 4

Large Intestine 4

Large Intestine 5

Triple Warmer 4

Triple Warmer 5

Triple Warmer 6

**Acupressure Points
on the Hand**

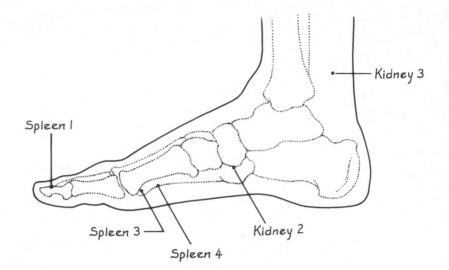

**Acupressure Points
on the Inside of the Foot**

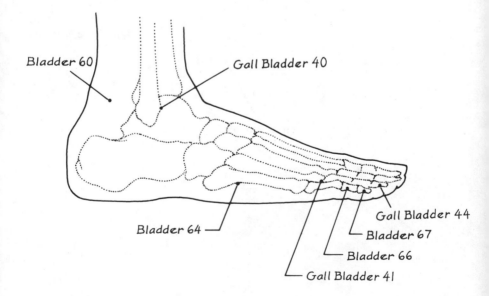

**Acupressure Points
on the Outside of the Foot**

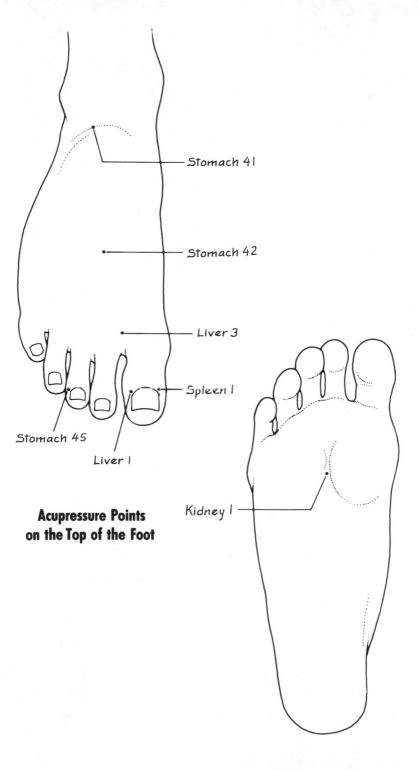

Stomach 41

Stomach 42

Liver 3

Spleen 1

Stomach 45

Liver 1

**Acupressure Points
on the Top of the Foot**

Kidney 1

**Acupressure Point
on the Bottom of the Foot**

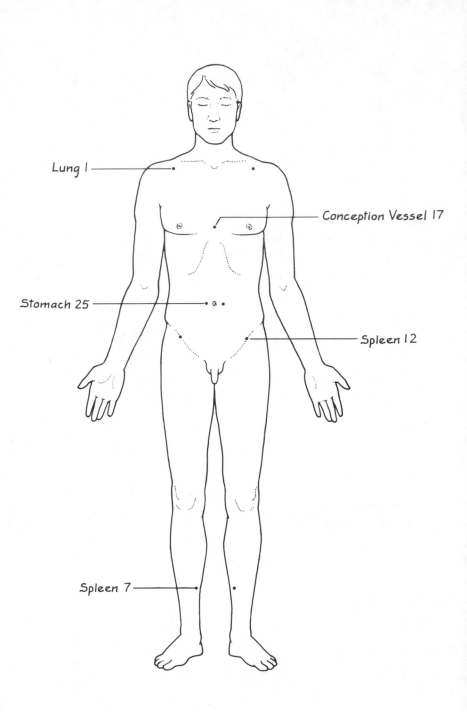

Lung 1

Conception Vessel 17

Stomach 25

Spleen 12

Spleen 7

**Golden Points
on the Front of the Body**

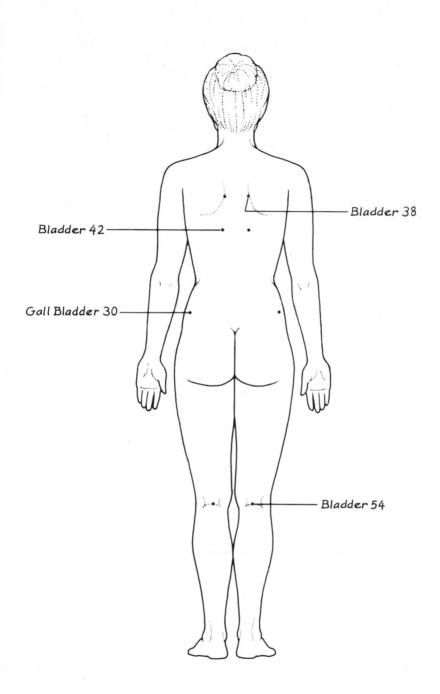

Bladder 38

Bladder 42

Gall Bladder 30

Bladder 54

**Golden Points
on the Back of the Body**

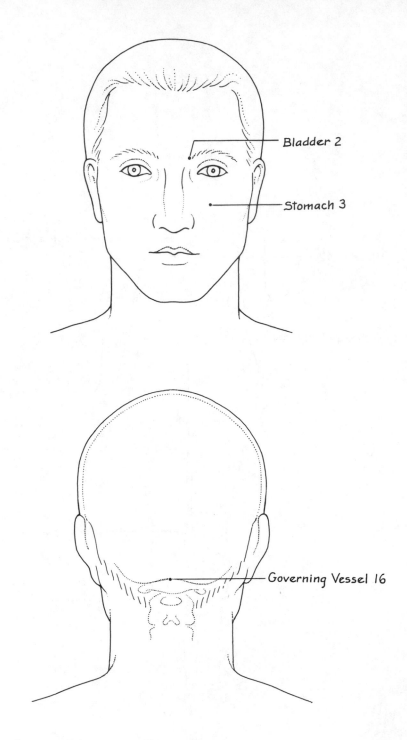

Bladder 2

Stomach 3

Governing Vessel 16

**Golden Points
on the Head Region**

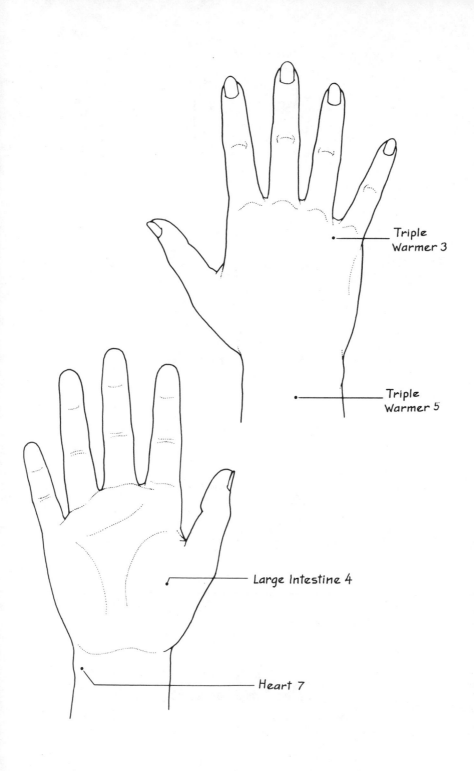

Triple
Warmer 3

Triple
Warmer 5

Large Intestine 4

Heart 7

**Golden Points
on the Hand**

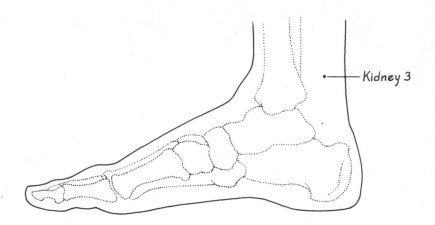

**Golden Point
on the Inside of the Foot**

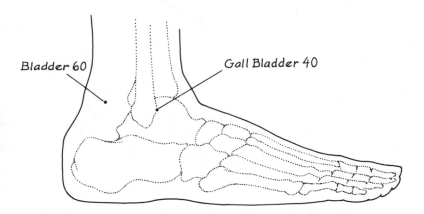

**Golden Points
on the Outside of the Foot**

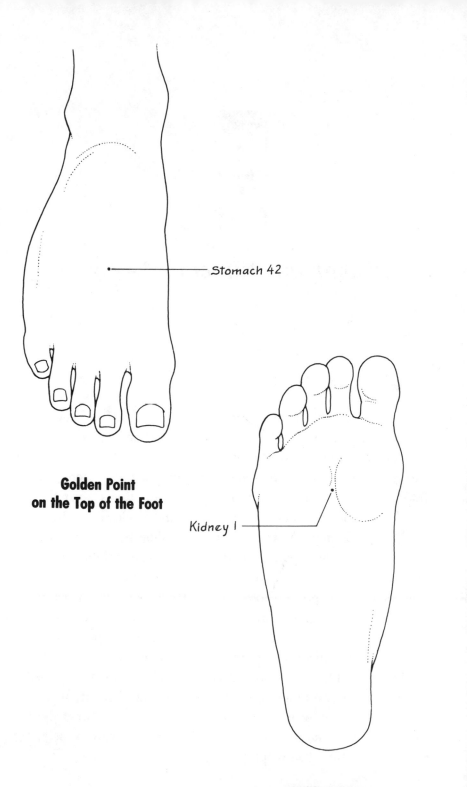

Stomach 42

**Golden Point
on the Top of the Foot**

Kidney 1

**Golden Point
on the Bottom of the Foot**

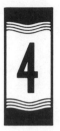

Common Ailments A-Z

Abrasions (Scrapes)

Abrasions occur when skin scrapes against a hard surface such as cement. This breaks the skin's top layers, and stings. Pieces of gravel or dirt may cling to the skin.

Run cold water over the scrape to remove bacteria-laden grit. Wrap a piece of ice in a clean cloth, and press this against the wound to numb the pain. When the wound is clean and bandaged, press Golden Points to promote healing by relaxing the muscles around the wound. Tight, tense muscles inhibit blood flow, limiting the supply of red blood cells and nutrients to the healing skin. If the point is located directly on the wound, avoid it. Direct finger pressure may cause pain and tissue damage. Choose another point or stimulate circulation by gently massaging the muscles surrounding the wound. Pure aloe vera gel, available in health food stores, soothes broken skin. It is also thought to promote tissue healing. For maximum benefit, apply aloe vera gel to the wound three to six times a day. Protect the broken skin from harmful bacteria by covering it with a clean bandage every time you reapply the gel.

Acne

Acne, an outbreak of reddish pimples and blackheads on the skin surface, is associated with adolescence and Premenstrual Syndrome. Acne also appears in response to stress, and may be caused by food or medications, or a combination of these, regardless of age or sex.

Pimples and blackheads occur when skin follicles become clogged with oil and infected by skin bacteria. Eliminate acne and prevent its recurrence by cleansing and toning your skin, avoiding fatty foods, and pressing acupressure points to stimulate circulation and improve your body's ability to eliminate wastes. Chinese medical practitioners view acne as an elimination problem caused by insufficient energy in the Large Intestine meridian. Strengthen the Large Intestine and release facial tension, which blocks circulation, by pressing four or more of these points every day: Large Intestine 1, 4 (do not use 4 in pregnancy), 11, 20, Bladder 2, Stomach 3 and 6, Triple Warmer 23, and Liver 3.

Supplement your acupressure points with a weekly rose clay mask to cleanse skin deeply and provide nutrients. You can also use brewer's yeast as a mask, or take it internally. This niacin-rich food supplement is available in health food stores. Jenny found that three brewer's yeast tablets per day controlled her acne breakouts.

Brewer's yeast has been known to increase the itching and burning symptoms of yeast infections.

Altitude Sickness

Altitude sickness sometimes occurs when hikers and travelers ascend too rapidly. Its symptoms include nausea, vomiting, headache, poor appetite, and insomnia. Altitude sickness seldom lasts longer than forty-eight hours. It can usually be minimized or prevented by a slow and gradual ascent. For example, backpackers headed for high country can drive to their start-off point, then sleep beside the car the night before their climb. Plan ahead to avoid altitude sickness. Use maps and tourist guides to set realistic goals for daily travel.

If altitude sickness strikes, however, you can use acupressure to ease its symptoms. To relieve nausea press Stomach 25 and 42 and Spleen 4; for dizziness press Stomach 36 (do not use in pregnancy), Stomach 42, and Kidney 3; for fatigue press Kidney 1 (do not use in pregnancy), Kidney 3, Lung 1, Lung 2, and Conception Vessel 17. Also see the entries for Fatigue, page 65, Insomnia, page 77, and Stomach/Abdominal Discomfort, page 94.

Anal Fissure

If you find blood on your underwear, you may have a break in your anal membrane. This could be caused by straining too hard when you have a bowel movement (see Constipation, page 57), hemorrhoids (see Hemorrhoids, page 71), or skin dryness (see Chapped Skin, page 52). If you have anal sexual contact, your partner may be too rough, or may not use sufficient lubrication. Anal injury sometimes occurs as the result of sexual assault as well.

Anal fissures are not usually painful unless they remain untreated and become infected. Keep your rectal area clean with water and glycerine soap (see Resources, page 131), washing every time you have a bowel movement. Press Spleen 12, Bladder 48, Governing Vessel 2, and Conception Vessel 2 to stimulate healing circulation.

Anxiety

Anxiety is an emotional response to stress. It may last for a few moments, several hours or days, or it may be a chronic problem. Anxiety often stimulates the appearance of physical symptoms, including perspiration and trembling. It almost always causes shallow breathing, and it makes thinking or speaking difficult.

Anxiety focuses your attention on a negative future possibility rather than keeping your full attention in the present. If you are frequently anxious, you may find yourself apologizing constantly, being unable to relax, and constantly angling for reassurance from other people. Chronic, omnipresent anxiety often seems to have no particular focus.

Asian medical practitioners associate anxiety with an imbalanced Spleen and Stomach energy, observing that an Earth imbalance can make you worried and forgetful as well as impair your perspective. You can press acupressure points to calm yourself, promote deep, relaxed breathing, and bring yourself into the present. Classic points for anxiety relief are Stomach 42, Spleen 3, Lung 1 and 2, Heart 5 and 7, and Pericardium 5. Concentrating on point location helps focus your attention, which in turn makes it easier for you to acknowledge your anxiety, identify the circumstances that inspired your feelings, and deal with them constructively. Mark pressed Stomach 42 and Spleen 3 while he sat in a dentist's waiting room, then pressed Heart 5 to calm himself while she capped a molar. He reported, "I actually felt relaxed after the dentist! I even felt okay enough to go back to work after the appointment."

For maximum benefit, supplement acupressure points with the following calming meditation. You may find it helpful to read this into a tape recorder and play it back when you need to relax.

A CALMING MEDITATION

Stand or sit comfortably. Inhale. Imagine that you are inhaling a golden light. Draw it deeply into your lungs. Now exhale. See yourself expelling a cloud of gray, stagnant air. Let the exhalation complete itself before you inhale again. Repeat until you feel calmer.

Now bring your attention to your feet. Feel the way your feet connect with the floor or the earth. Feel the earth supporting you.

Again, breathe slowly and deeply until your anxiety symptoms pass.

Asthma

Asthma attacks are characterized by wheezing, breathing difficulty, and chest oppression. Laurel described it this way: "It's like there's this big stone on my chest, and it's crushing my breath." These are frightening sensations for the sufferers and for the people around them.

Asthma attacks often begin very suddenly, in response to stress, allergens, or minor respiratory infections such as colds. When the body perceives a threat from these stimuli, it produces antibodies, substances that neutralize toxins. This reaction ultimately causes cells to release mucus and other fluids that contract the bronchial walls and narrow the breathing passage. This drastically reduces the lungs' oxygen supply.

Relaxation minimizes bronchial wall constriction, widens the air passage, and makes breathing easier. You can use affirmations, acupressure, and other techniques like the Calming Meditation on page 43 for a relaxing effect. At the first sign of an asthma attack, silently repeat these affirmations:

> I breathe deeply and easily.
> I feel calm and safe.
> My breath is strong and even.

Continue these affirmations while you press Lung 1 and 2, Conception Vessel 17, and Bladder 38. Continue pressing until your symptoms abate and repeat points which seem particularly helpful.

Back Pain and Tension

Back pain typically begins with muscle or ligament fatigue and tension that results from poor posture, a lack of exercise, or the frequent use of an uncomfortable chair, desk, or workbench. It can also occur if you omit warm-up and cool-down stretches in an exercise routine, or if you habitually sit for most of the day. PMS sufferers sometimes experience lower back pain during the two weeks prior to menstruation.

Spinal discomfort may also be due to a disc problem. Discs are the cushiony sacks between your vertebrae that pad these spinal bones. They may crack, chip, or protrude if the vertebrae are misaligned. Disc problems also result from chronic stress in the ligaments that keep the vertebrae together. For deep back pain, consult a doctor or chiropractor who can order X rays to identify fracture, dislocation, or other bone damage.

Relieve your aching back with tension reducing acupressure, stretching, and hot compresses. Ask a friend to press Governing Vessel 2 and 4 and Bladder 38, 45, and 48, or use an old, soft tennis ball for points you cannot reach. Place the ball beneath the point and ease onto it slowly and gently, supporting yourself on your elbows. Supplement your acupressure with stretching for maximum tension relief. Practice the stretches shown on page 129 at least once every day to relieve back pain and stiffness and prevent its recurrence. Also see the entry for Joint Pain and Stiffness, page 78.

Balanitis (Foreskin Inflammation)

Balanitis is a painful inflammation of the foreskin and penis in an uncircumcised male. Bacteria trapped beneath the foreskin or an abrasive injury are the main causes. If you have balanitis, it stings when you urinate, and there may be a discharge from the penis. There are also flulike symptoms of chills, fever, and enlarged lymph glands in the groin area (see the entries for Influenza, page 75, and Fever, page 66). Balanitis symptoms should be checked by a doctor since they approximate some sexually transmitted diseases.

Rest in bed until your temperature returns to normal and your energy returns. Relieve balanitis discomfort by pressing Conception Vessel 2 and 3 for at least five minutes each. Then supplement your acupressure with warm (not hot!) gingerroot compresses. Peel and chop about a tablespoonful of fresh gingerroot (available in most supermarkets and health food stores), wrap it in a clean square of unbleached muslin, and pour hot water over it. When this compress is cool enough to touch, push the foreskin back and place it on your penis. You may also find it comforting to place a larger compress on your lower back, over your kidneys.

You can help prevent a recurrence by keeping the area beneath your foreskin very clean, and by strengthening the meridians that govern genital health. Asian physicians regard balanitis and other genital problems as a symptom of low energy in the Water meridians. In addition to using acupressure for instant relief during the acute stage, press at least one of these points daily: Kidney 1, Kidney 3, Kidney 7, Kidney 11, Bladder 64, Conception Vessel 2, Governing Vessel 14. To prevent a recurrence continue this daily practice for one month after your symptoms disappear. Every third day, press Spleen 3, Stomach 42, and Heart 7 to strengthen Fire and Earth; these meridians support Water in caring for your reproductive system.

Bed-wetting

See Urinary Incontinence, page 98.

Bee Stings

See Insect Stings, page 76.

Bladder Symptoms

Bladder symptoms typically include frequent and painful urination. An inflamed bladder has a smaller volume and nearly always feels full. Cystitis, a common bladder infection, usually produces traces of blood in the urine. See a doctor if your symptoms include fever, extreme fatigue, and backache.

Men with venereal disease almost always have bladder symptoms. Therefore, it is essential for men with urinary discomfort to refrain from sexual contact until tested by an M.D.

Doctors typically encourage patients with bladder infections to increase fluid intake. Frequent urination cleanses the bladder and stops bacteria reproduction. Replace your chemically dyed toilet paper with a plain white brand, as you could be sensitive to certain dyes. (See Resources, page 131.)

Asian medical practitioners use acupressure points to stimulate urination and tone the Kidney and Bladder meridians, which regulate the urinary system. During a bout with bladder symptoms, press two or more of these points three times per day: Bladder 60, 64, 66, and 67 and Kidney 3 and 8.

Avoid coffee, black tea, and alcohol, all of which contain potential bladder irritants. Drink plenty of distilled water, cranberry juice (check the label to make sure it's free of additives), and cornsilk tea. This home remedy is made by steeping one teaspoon of cornsilk (inside the cornhusk) in one cup of boiling water until it is cool enough to drink. Consume at least three cups per day until your symptoms disappear.

To help prevent a recurrence, continue pressing these points for two weeks after your symptoms disappear.

Bleeding

Wound bleeding is controlled by strong, direct hand pressure. Place a sterile gauze pad or clean cloth over the wound, then press against it with your entire hand. If a pad or cloth is unavailable, apply your hand to the wound. Hold firmly for three or more minutes until the bleeding has ceased. Alternatively, you can apply a sterile gauze pad to an arm or leg wound and loosely wind an ace bandage around the limb. Make sure it's loose enough to permit circulation.

Do not improvise a tourniquet; these tight bandages can cause nerve and blood vessel damage.

Substantial bleeding is a medical emergency that requires prompt attention at a doctor's office or an emergency room.

Blisters

Blisters are part of the healing process of second- and third-degree burns. They can also be caused by friction, when the skin is repeatedly rubbed across underlying tissues. This digs a cleft in the mid-portion of the epidermis, the skin's top layer. The cleft fills with fluid. Blisters can also be caused by stiff shoe leather rubbing against a foot. (Wear new footwear for an hour or two each day with socks or stockings until the leather softens.)

Blisters should be covered, particularly if the skin is broken, as the open wound is prone to infection. Press Golden Points around the bandage to relieve pain and stimulate circulation. Apply aloe vera or a room temperature marigold poultice, then cover the blister with a clean bandage; repeat this at least three times a day. You can further protect the blister by covering the bandage with moleskin, a thick, clothlike skin protector available in camping supply stores.

Boils

A boil looks like a swollen red pimple with a white top. It is actually a bacterial infection. When hair follicles are plugged with oil, they become breeding grounds for bacteria. The resulting infection produces a swelling that is painful if it presses a nerve ending. You should see your doctor if the boil is near your nostrils or inside your ear, since this gives the infection easy access to the brain. If you are a nursing mother, your obstetrician should be consulted about boils on your breasts.

Prevent further infection by washing the boil and surrounding skin at least four times daily, using warm water and glycerine soap. Between washings apply a hot washcloth directly to the boil. The warm heat increases blood flow. This draws nutrients and antibodies to counteract the bacterial infection. Press the Golden Points nearest the boil to ease the muscular tension that inhibits circulation.

For painful or persistent boils, alternate hot compresses and acupressure with a green-clay paste. Use hot water to prepare the clay. Apply it directly to the boil and allow it to dry before rinsing it off. Repeat at least twice a day until the boil disappears.

Breathing Difficulties

Breathing difficulties may result from colds and other respiratory problems like asthma. Toxic substances such as air pollution often cause labored breathing. Some people hyperventilate or breathe too shallowly when they are anxious and upset.

Whether or not there are obvious causes (such as a toxic substance) present, severe breathing difficulty can be the first stage of a medical emergency. (See the entries for Insect Stings, page 76, and A Medical Emergency, page 108.)

The first step in treating breathing difficulties is to remove yourself from the potential problem. Go outside to clean, fresh air and lie down if possible. Lie quietly while you press Lung 1 and 2, Conception Vessel 17, and Bladder 38.

Also see the entries for Asthma, page 44, Colds and Bronchitis, page 54, Hay Fever, page 69, Nasal Congestion, page 84, and Smoke Inhalation, page 93.

Bruises

A bruise results from a blow to the skin surface. The skin doesn't break, but small blood vessels beneath the skin's surface are lacerated, which permits blood to escape into the surrounding skin tissue. This is what causes discoloration. Bruises are painful and are tender to the touch.

As soon as you bump yourself, press the Golden Point nearest the injury site. Then massage and press the surrounding skin area to stimulate circulation. If you have ice handy, press it against the painful area to anesthetize it and minimize discoloration.

Bruxism (Tooth Grinding)

Habitual tooth clenching and grinding, or bruxism, is a stress response that leads to headache, facial tension, and pain. Untreated chronic bruxism can cause tooth degeneration and dysfunction of the temporomandibular joint (this enables you to open and shut your mouth).

Bruxism sufferers can benefit from acupressure tension relief. Pressing Stomach 3, 5, and 6, Large Intestine 20, Triple Warmer 23 (press all of these on both sides of your face), Governing Vessel 24, Conception Vessel 17 and 24, and the extra point beneath the nose trains your muscles to release jaw tension and stress. Press at least three points during the day and three more before going to sleep at night. You should feel some decrease in tension after two weeks of faithfully pressing points. This effect is enhanced when you use supplementary techniques such as visualization (see A Calming Meditation on page 43) and nutritional aids.

Calcium and magnesium in combination, sometimes marketed as dolomite, is a natural muscle relaxant. This nutrient combination is readily available in pharmacies and health food stores. Adults usually add 900 to 1200 milligrams per day to their diets. Add it to your diet gradually to prevent constipation, a common side effect. Take your calcium and magnesium combination every other day for two weeks, two out of three days for another two weeks, then use it daily.

Burns

There are three types of heat injuries classified by severity. *First-degree burns* affect only the top layer of the skin, producing redness, mild pain, and swelling. These burns are typically produced by minor accidents such as brushing against a hot cooking pot or staying in the sun too long. *Second-degree burns* strike more deeply, causing blisters (don't break these open), sharp pain, and swelling; these symptoms last for several days. Touching the skin to boiling water or a heating coil will usually cause second-degree burns.

Third-degree burns injure all skin layers and require immediate attention at a doctor's office or an emergency room. These raw whitish burns are caused by prolonged exposure to flame. Many third-degree burn patients were trapped in a burning building or automobile.

The first step in burn treatment is to put out or remove the heat source. Douse the flames of a small fire (such as a grease fire in a frying pan) or move away from the fire and telephone for emergency assistance. Unplug the source of an electrical fire if you can get to the socket without compromising your safety.

Remove heat-retaining jewelry and clothing from the burned skin, and run cold water over it. This washes out cloth fragments and eases the sting. If pain persists, apply an ice pack.

Douse the burn with aloe vera gel. For the maximum benefit, apply the gel as frequently as every thirty minutes. Press Golden Points near the burned area at least three times daily to stimulate circulation.

Keep the burn clean and covered with a bandage.

Bursitis

See Joint Pain and Stiffness, page 78.

Calluses and Corns

Calluses and corns are small segments of thickened, hardened skin, resulting from continual rubbing and pressing. Corns appear on the feet and are similar to warts, except that they are sensitive to touch. Calluses are usually painless although they sometimes crack open. This wound should be cleaned, dabbed with aloe vera gel, and bandaged to keep out harmful bacteria.

Shrink corns and calluses with a daily green-clay poultice. This softens the skin and stimulates surface circulation. While you wait for the poultice to dry, massage the area with your fingertips and press Golden Points. This also increases healing circulation.

Canker Sores

Canker sores are small painful wounds of the mucous membranes inside your mouth. You typically get them if you're eating too much sugar or feel chronically stressed. Chinese physicians treat canker sores by strengthening the Small Intestine and Liver meridians, which help us to retain nutrients and discard potentially harmful substances from food. Press Liver 3, and Small Intestine 4 and 10 (10 is not used in pregnancy) twice daily until your canker sores disappear.

If the sores persist, supplement your acupressure points with echinacea mouthwash. Steep two tablespoons of the dried herb in one cup of boiling water until it is cool enough to drink. Take a mouthful of this tea and hold it against the canker sore for three to five minutes. Then swallow. Repeat the process until you've swallowed the whole cup. The echinacea mouthwash is taken three or four times a day until the canker sores disappear.

Chapped Skin

Chapped skin is red, dry, and sometimes painful. It is caused by excessive exposure to wind and sun. Your skin can also become chapped when exposed to chemical irritants such as paint thinner.

Beauty professionals suggest that you avoid washing your face for half an hour before you go out into cold weather, since water contributes to chapping. You can also minimize chapping by protecting your skin with frequent applications of sunscreen and lip gloss. If you are prone to chapped skin, rub aloe vera gel and jojoba oil into the vulnerable areas each day. Massage these areas and press local Golden Points to stimulate circulation.

Claustrophobia

Claustrophobia is the fear of being enclosed in a small place, particularly for a lengthy period of time. Those who suffer claustrophobia often feel compelled to leave an enclosed space immediately. If this is impossible, many experience a rush of intense fear and physical symptoms such as dizziness, pounding heart, trembling, and vertigo. Some pace up and down when they do not feel they can leave an enclosed area. For example, Maggie's claustrophobia was initially diagnosed by her daughter's pediatrician, who came upon her pacing back and forth in an examining room.

Claustrophobia can cause great difficulty in school, work, and family life. John, age fifteen, was taken to an educational psychologist because of his "bad attitude" toward school. Fortunately, the counselor recognized his inability to pay attention and his habit of staring out the window as symptoms of claustrophobia and directed his parents to appropriate treatment.

When claustrophobia symptoms strike, try to relax. If you are able to leave the situation, do so. Look for a relaxing setting where you can press acupressure points and consciously slow your breathing. This eases panic symptoms and brings your attention to the present. Press at least three of the following points: Lung 1 and 2, Bladder 38, Heart 5, 7, 8, and 9, Pericardium 5 and 8, Spleen 3, and Stomach 42.

Also see the entries for Anxiety, page 42, and Panic, page 85.

Cold Hands and Feet

Chronically cold hands and feet usually result from inactive circulation and/or iron-deficiency anemia. This problem responds to a program of increased exercise, iron supplementation, and acupressure self-care.

Circulation is typically inhibited by lack of exercise and muscular tension. The acupressure treatment for cold hands and feet begins at the shoulders and pelvis, as tension in these areas limits blood flow to the extremities. Begin by easing into the stretches shown on pages 129, then press two or more of the following: Bladder 38, Small Intestine 10 (not to be used in pregnancy), Large Intestine 15, Gall Bladder 21, Triple Warmer 15 on the upper body, and Gall Bladder 30, Governing Vessel 2, and Bladder 54 for the legs and feet. Then press points which are directly on the extremities: Kidney 1 (not in pregnancy), Kidney 2, Kidney 3, Bladder 64, Stomach 40, Stomach 41, Spleen 3 for the upper body, and Triple Warmer 6, Pericardium 5, Pericardium 8 (not in pregnancy), Heart 8, Small Intestine 1, and Small Intestine 4 on the hands. Press these points twice daily for the maximum benefit.

Asian medical practitioners also treat poor circulation by activating the yang Fire meridians (Small Intestine and Triple Warmer) to increase heat and energy flow throughout the body. For long-term circulatory problems, Small Intestine 4 and Triple Warmer 3 are pressed each day. This is supplemented with gingerroot tea.

Gingerroot is available in the produce section of most supermarkets. Cut a piece approximately the size of your little finger, peel and dice it, then steep it in one cup of boiling water until the tea is cool enough to drink. Five cups per week is the standard dosage for adults. Children between the ages of four and twelve may be given three cups per week. Gingerroot should not be used during the first six months of pregnancy, since it is associated with excessive bleeding.

Colds and Bronchitis

Colds typically occur when you're fatigued and overstressed. In this state, your respiratory system develops an acidity which creates temperature and moisture levels hospitable to cold viruses. Your body responds to these invading viruses by increasing mucus production and blood flow, which brings antibodies and white cells in to attack the virus. This causes swollen, reddened mucus membranes in your throat and nasal passages. Other symptoms vary. They may include coughs, headache or sinus pain, and generalized muscular aches. A few cold sufferers (1 percent) run low fevers.

Bronchitis, an infection of the bronchial tubes in the upper part of the lungs, sometimes follows an untreated cold. This potentially serious disease is characterized by more intense cold symptoms that include deep fatigue and muscle aches. Your throat and lymph nodes are swollen, red, and painful. Since your bronchial tubes are also swollen, and partially blocked with mucus, breathing is difficult. You must rest in bed.

Many doctors will immediately prescribe antibiotics for bronchitis. If you elect to take them, ask your doctor to prescribe ampicillin. This antibiotic acts upon several types of bacteria, while some others will only affect one strain—possibly one that did not cause your bronchial infection. Antibiotics must be taken under an M.D.'s supervision. These powerful drugs will not be effective if you do not follow the directions on the label. For example, if you stop taking the medication as soon as you feel better, instead of completing the prescribed course, your symptoms will soon return. Some people are allergic to one or more types of antibiotic. Allergic reactions include rashes, dizziness, fainting, and convulsions.

You can press acupressure points while taking antibiotics, but avoid herbal remedies. The various ingredients may interact badly, causing unpleasant physical reactions (including allergylike symptoms). They may also cancel each other out in combination, thus rendering both substances chemically useless.

Acupressure points and herbal remedies relax you and relieve congestion. Press Lung 1, Lung 2, Bladder 48, and Conception Vessel 17. As these points release tension, let yourself cough deeply to loosen the mucus. A cough control center in your brain stimulates this important healing response to rid your body of mucus. Cough suppressants inhibit this, whether they are over the counter drugstore brands or are touted as natural remedies.

Herbal remedies are helpful. Chamomile tea soothes the throat and induces a restful sleep. Steep one teaspoon of the dried herb in one cup of boiling water until it is cool enough to drink. Chamomile is a mild tea that may be drunk freely (unless you are about to drive). Echinacea acts as an herbal antibiotic. Research suggests that echinacea blocks infection by reinforcing the white blood cells and the hyaluronidase system, which binds cells together and forms a barrier against harmful bacteria. To make echinacea tea, steep one teaspoon of the dried herb in one cup of boiling water until it is cool enough to drink. Take up to three cups per day for ten days.

Antibiotics often stimulate monilia, or yeast growth, causing an itching and burning sensation in your genital area. If you are vulnerable to yeast infections, it may help you to begin acupressure self-treatment the same day you start a course of antibiotics. (See entry for Monilia, page 83.)

Also see entries for Hay Fever, page 69, Fatigue, page 65, and Pharyngitis, page 87.

Conjunctivitis (Pinkeye)

Pinkeye is the common name for conjunctivitis, a bacterial or viral infection of the mucosal membrane in the eye. Its symptoms are itching, tears, and a sticky discharge. Occasionally there is pain and swelling. Untreated pinkeye typically lasts for ten to fourteen days. Doctors prescribe antibiotic ointments or drops for bacterial conjunctivitis. Viral conjunctivitis does not respond to antibiotic therapy.

If you have conjunctivitis, be careful to use only your own washcloth and towel. Pinkeye is extremely infectious. Don't share cosmetics, and wash your hands with soap and water immediately after touching your eyes.

Acupressure points and goldenseal herb relieve the itching and swelling. Press Liver 3 (used by Chinese physicians for infections and allergic reactions) and Spleen 7 for itching. Continue with Bladder 1 and 2, Gall Bladder 1, and Stomach 1. Remember to wash your hands when you're finished!

Supplement your acupressure points with a goldenseal eyewash. (This herb should not be used during pregnancy.) Brew a strong pot of goldenseal tea (two teaspoons of the powdered herb to each cup of boiling water). Let it cool, then splash it on your eyes throughout the day. Alternatively, soak a clean piece of unbleached muslin in the teapot and place it over your eyes while you lie down to rest. Throw away the muslin when you're finished.

For maximum relief, apply acupressure points and goldenseal eyewash at least three times a day until your pinkeye is healed.

Constipation

Constipation is the temporary cessation of bowel movements. The intestinal motion that propels stools through the intestines is sometimes disrupted by stress or dietary changes. Calcium and iron supplements may have a binding effect if they are added to your diet suddenly. Emotional upset also causes the muscular intestinal walls to clench, thus inhibiting waste movement.

Combine a program of acupressure, diet, and exercise to relieve constipation. Acupressure's relaxing effect relieves clenched intestinal muscles. Press Large Intestine 4 (not to be used in pregnancy), Large Intestine 11, and Conception Vessel 3 to ease intestinal tension and stimulate intestinal peristalsis. If you suspect your constipation is stress related, begin reducing stress by pressing these three points each day and review the entry for Anxiety, page 42.

Doctors typically suggest that patients suffering from constipation drink more water, increase their fiber intake by eating fresh fruits and vegetables every day, and exercise. (Exercise is a well-known laxative.)

Contact Dermatitis (Rash)

Rashes are composed of small itchy blisters on a red background. They commonly appear in response to irritants like cosmetics, jewelry, or detergents. You may get a heat rash in the armpit or groin if you wear tight clothing, especially in humid weather, or neglect to dry the area thoroughly after bathing. Some people suffer from rashes during stressful periods.

Wash the rash frequently with water and additive-free soap. (See Resources, page 131.) This aids in eliminating harmful bacteria, which can enter your body through the skin eruption. If you rub or scratch the rash you can expect it to linger, as well as to increase in size. Avoid spreading the rash by washing your hands thoroughly each time you touch it.

Press Spleen 7 at least three times daily to relieve the itching and heat. A paste of dried goldenseal herb also relieves the itching. If the rash is widespread, pour a half-cup of goldenseal into a warm bath. (Goldenseal herb should not be used during pregnancy.)

When the substance that caused it is identified and banished, rashes typically disappear within twenty-four hours. Asian medical practitioners believe that frequent bouts with contact dermatitis result from a weakened liver, since it plays an important role in filtering harmful materials from your body. They treat people with frequent rashes by pressing Liver 3, a traditional toner.

Also see Jock Rot, page 77.

Cramps

A cramp is a sharp, painful muscular contraction that has several possible causes. You may experience a cramp in any part of your body that remains too long in an uncomfortable position. Heat cramps result from a failure to replace the fluids lost by sweating during vigorous exercise. Many women suffer painful uterine contractions during menstrual periods (see Menstrual Cramps, page 83).

Acupressure relieves cramp pain by relaxing muscles. Use strong, direct pressure on the Golden Point nearest the muscle pain. Press the point until the pain is completely relieved (this may take from six to ten minutes for deep muscle spasms), then massage the muscles to increase circulation and prevent a recurrence.

You can take steps to prevent excessive heat loss during exercise. Drink enough water to keep your body weight constant. You can carry a canteen during workouts and take a sip every time your mouth feels dry. Salt tablets help you retain fluid during heavy training (do not use these if you have hypertension). A diet that includes at least four fresh fruit and vegetable servings per day provides you with nutrients that minimize heat cramping.

Depression

Depression is a complex emotional state that typically includes feelings of hopelessness, lack of control, and low self-esteem. It often stimulates unpleasant physical symptoms that include fatigue, substance addictions, and vulnerability to disease. Depression sometimes results from hormonal changes following surgery or childbirth; it can be aggravated when the nervous system is stressed by a sugar- and fat-laden diet and a lack of exercise. The specific cause should be identified and treated, sometimes in consultation with a mental health professional. If you are depressed for longer than a week, have recurring thoughts of suicide, or a chronic feeling of worthlessness, psychiatric care is necessary; prescription drug therapy is recommended in some cases.

Professional opinions vary with regard to physical and psychological origins. Janice Phelps, M.D., director of the Alternatives in Medicine Clinic in Seattle, believes that low endorphin production causes depression. Her treatment utilizes holistic techniques that stimulate endorphin production. Others prefer behavior-oriented therapies. Shoma Morita, a Japanese psychiatrist, developed his Constructive Living therapy, which teaches that feelings result from behavior. Constructive Living is accomplishment oriented, with an emphasis on feeding self-worth by involvement with outside activities such as sports, the arts, or social action.

Several of my acupressure clients found that their mild depression was relieved with self-care that combined mental techniques, positive action, and pressing points. Allison was encouraged to press acupressure points each day and to return to the Caribbean dance classes she had given up earlier. The exercise raised her spirits and relieved muscular tension. She also made friends in her dance class. Mark combined acupressure with a change of diet, substituting regular meals for the coffee and candy he nibbled throughout the day. Soon he felt calmer, more energetic, and strong enough to tackle his underlying problems, which included low self-esteem and a lack of connection with others. He eventually resolved these by volunteering at a local hospice. Mark found that helping terminally ill patients with daily tasks increased his self-esteem "because I am giving my time and energy to something that really matters, making their lives a little easier."

Acupressure points for depression are Heart 5, 7, 8, 9, Pericardium 8 (not to be used in pregnancy), Stomach 40, Stomach 45 (not to be used in pregnancy), Kidney 1 (also not to be used in pregnancy), Lung 1, Lung 2, and Large Intestine 1.

Diarrhea

Diarrhea is a digestive condition that causes food to pass through your system quickly without giving you much nutritive value. Its causes include viral infections, food poisoning, and bacterial dysentery (Montezuma's Revenge) spread via unwashed fruits and vegetables. Diarrhea may also occur in response to stress. It is occasionally accompanied by cramping (see the entries for Cramps, page 58, and Stomach/Abdominal Discomfort, page 94).

Acupressure clients found that Stomach 25 and Bladder 48 relieved diarrhea symptoms. Press these two points for at least five minutes, every half hour, until the diarrhea is relieved.

Supplement these points with plenty of water or mint teas to replace fluids lost in watery bowel movements. Natural healing systems encourage diarrhea sufferers to avoid dairy products, sugary foods, and raw produce for several days, as these food substances are regarded as colon irritants. Children under two years of age are customarily given weak peppermint tea and water in place of milk.

Dry Eyes

Dry eyes burn, feel itchy and gritty, and tire easily. Insufficient eye lubrication can result from wind exposure, collagen vascular diseases such as rheumatoid arthritis and Sjogren's Syndrome, antihistamines, and antidepressants. It sometimes follows a bout with conjunctivitis (see the entry for Conjunctivitis, page 56), or exposure to polluted air. Doctors typically prescribe artificial teardrops and ointments for dry eyes. Some people are sensitive to the preservatives in these substances and experience further irritation.

You can press acupressure points to relieve eye dryness. Bladder 1 and 2 and Gall Bladder 1 relieve tension in the muscles surrounding the eyes and stimulate tearing. These are traditional tonic points for the Wood meridians, which govern eyesight. Press these points on both sides of the face for relief, repeating as needed.

Ear Discomfort

Ear discomfort and pain can be caused by a blockage or infection. If your hearing seems less keen than usual, and your ears feel full, the ear canal may be blocked by a buildup of cerumen (earwax). Use an irrigating syringe to squirt a mixture of mild liquid soap and water into the ear. *Do not attempt to dig the wax out of your ear!*

When you insert any object into the ear canal, you risk severe damage to the eardrum.

Other symptoms may include painful swelling, itching, and ear discharge, which can indicate an ear infection. These are sometimes caused by fungus and bacteria living in lakes, ponds, and swimming pools. Your doctor will identify the type of infection and prescribe the appropriate antibiotic.

After appropriate medical treatment, acupressure points relieve the pain and itching. Acupressure practitioners work to prevent a recurrence by toning the Water meridians, which are associated with hearing. Angela pressed Small Intestine 4 to relieve her young son's earache, which was caused by a recurrent inner ear infection. When he recovered, she made a game of pressing Kidney 1 (not to be used on pregnant women) and Bladder 64 during his nightly bath. About six weeks after she began this treatment, he suffered a final ear infection. This resolved quickly and did not return.

Eczema

Eczema is an itchy, scaly skin rash. Eczema looks and feels like some forms of contact dermatitis, but it is more swollen. Sometimes a patch of eczema will blister and ooze over with yellowish pus. It most commonly appears on the face, scalp, neck, and in the folds of the elbows and knees. Eczema appears in response to allergens or stress in susceptible adults and children.

Wash eczema frequently with water, glycerine soap (see Resources, page 131). Instead of using a washcloth, scrub the patch gently with paper towels. Throw them away when you're finished. This will help keep the eczema from spreading. Instead of rubbing or scratching, press Spleen 7 to relieve itching, and douse the eczema with soothing aloe vera gel. You will avoid spreading the rash if you wash your hands thoroughly after each contact.

Also see the entries for Chapped Skin, page 52, Contact Dermatitis, page 58, and Psoriasis, page 90.

Epididymitis (Scrotum Inflammation and Infection)

Epididymitis is an infection that produces a swollen, hardened testicle. This feels very sensitive, sometimes with burning pain. Epididymitis is frequently a complication of injury, prostate, or urinary tract infection. (See the entries for Bladder Symptoms, page 46, Prostate Symptoms, page 90, and Testicle Torsion, page 97.) Fever is usually part of epididymitis, and you feel achy and fatigued. (See the entry for Fever, page 66.) Rest in bed until your temperature returns to normal.

Press Conception Vessel 2 and 3, and make a gingerroot compress to relieve the immediate discomfort. Peel and chop about a tablespoonful of fresh gingerroot (available in most supermarkets and health food stores), wrap it in a clean square of unbleached muslin, and pour hot water over it. When this compress is cool enough to touch, set it on the swollen testicle. You may also find it comforting to place a larger compress on your lower back, over your kidneys.

Press Liver 3, Kidney 1 and 3, Bladder 64, and Conception Vessel 6 twice each day until your symptoms disappear. Help prevent a recurrence by pressing these points daily for two weeks thereafter.

Doctors usually treat epididymitis with antibiotics, and suggest sexual abstinence for a month after the symptoms disappear, which is protection against further infection.

Excessive Perspiration

Excessive perspiration can have many causes. It is often the result of nervousness or anxiety (see the entries for Anxiety, page 42, and Panic, page 85). It can also be a side effect of some medications. If you are taking a prescription medication, be sure to notify your doctor if you experience this unpleasant side effect.

Asian health practitioners regard excess perspiration as a symptom of too much heat within the body. They treat Bladder 64 and 66 and Kidney 3 and 8 to strengthen the cooling Water meridians and dampen the heat. Press these points for at least two minutes each, three times daily, until the condition is relieved.

Eyestrain

Overworked eyes feel tired and achy, and make it difficult to read or perform detail work. In severe cases of eyestrain, tiny red blood vessels are seen in the whites of the eyes.

Prevent eyestrain by using adequate light for detail work such as office tasks or technical equipment repair. Replace weak light bulbs promptly. You might try a strong "daylight bulb," designed to replicate outdoor light. These can be purchased at lighting and art supply stores. If you frequently work at a computer terminal, minimize eye stress by keeping the screen clean, and arrange your workload so that you perform an alternate task (or take a break) every hour.

You can further prevent and relieve eyestrain with yogic eye exercises (described below) and acupressure points that strengthen eye muscles and improve circulation.

STRENGTHEN YOUR EYES

1. *Keeping your chin still, raise your eyes all the way upward (strain slightly). Hold them all the way up and count to five.*
2. *Look downward, as far as you can, without moving your chin up or down. Hold your eyes in position and count to five.*
3. *Raise and lower your eyes quickly ten times. Move them as fast as you can.*
4. *Look all the way to the right and hold your eyes there for five counts. Repeat on the left. Then flash your eyes from right to left, pressing as far as you can to each side.*
5. *Roll your eyes in both directions. Try to make complete circles.*

Fainting

Fainting is a temporary loss of consciousness, usually preceded by dizziness and weakness. It is typically caused by a sudden drop in blood pressure that results from blood loss, shock, or exhaustion; it also indicates sunstroke.

If you suddenly feel weak, sit or lie down at once; you can injure yourself if you fall during a faint. Drivers should pull over to the side of the road and turn off the engine until they've recovered. Elevate your feet and drink plenty of cool water.

If someone near you faints, lay him or her down, out of direct sunlight and prop up the feet. When they regain consciousness, give water.

Asian practitioners use strong, abrupt pressure on Kidney 1 (not to be used in pregnancy) to restore consciousness (its nickname is Corpse Revival). Once the fainter is awake, he is likely to feel weak, dizzy, and nauseated. Keep him quiet and press the points for Fatigue, page 65, and Stomach/Abdominal Discomfort, page 94.

Fatigue

Fatigue is a signal to relax and renew your energy.

You can cope with moderate fatigue by balancing productive periods with rest and recreation. However, fatigue can be excessive and even chronic in some cases. Low energy levels can have

---

"THERE'S SOMETHING IN MY EYE"

Press Bladder 1 when there's something in the eye that shouldn't be there. It produces tears to speed expulsion of irritating foreign bodies such as dust, grit, or a stuck contact lense.

---

physical and psychological origins. If you are constantly tired, overwork may not be the problem.

Chronic, unacknowledged stress is a great fatiguer. Kyra Nichols, a principal dancer in the New York City Ballet, says that relaxation is the cornerstone of her legendary stamina. She taught herself to work without negative mental chatter; this freed her to dance naturally, without fatigue-producing tension.

Chronic fatigue is also a symptom of organic diseases including iron-deficiency anemia, urinary disorders, and hypoglycemia (low blood sugar), all of which are confirmed by laboratory tests. Your diet could also be a culprit. An unbalanced, sugar-heavy diet denies you the nutrients your body needs to manufacture energy. Some practitioners also suggest that fatigue-prone clients keep their blood sugar raised with small meals every two to three hours. For the maximum benefit, choose fibrous foods like fruit, vegetable, and whole-grain bread products that contain few (if any) sweeteners. These foods are digested slowly, supplying a continual flow of energy.

Asian medical practitioners look to the kidneys, the reserve energy storehouse, when patients complain of fatigue. Prolonged stress or poor health habits deplete energy resources. The kidneys are toned with the acupressure points Kidney 1 (not to be used in pregnancy), 3, 11, and 22. Stomach 36, traditionally known as Three More Miles, is also used for quick fatigue relief. This treatment is supplemented with daily kidney massage. Make loose fists and vigorously rub your lower back. It feels good to do this in the shower, with water running down your back.

Fever

Fever is a temperature elevation that occurs when harmful bacteria or viruses invade your body, stimulating heat-producing pyrogens. Your body responds by sweating to cool itself. Childhood fevers are typically associated with respiratory infection, although they also signal urinary tract infections in prepubescent girls. An infant younger than one month should promptly be examined by a doctor if his rectal temperature is higher than 100 degrees Fahrenheit.

Doctors consider that fever is present in older children and adults when the temperature is 100 degrees Fahrenheit by mouth. Medical attention is necessary if your temperature remains higher than 102 degrees for a day or more. Rest in bed and press acupressure points until your temperature returns to normal.

Bladder 66 and Kidney 8 are the traditional points for reducing fever. These are supplemented by Pericardium 7, Triple Warmer 4 (not to be used in pregnancy), Heart 7, and Small Intestine 4, which balance the energy in the Fire meridians. You can also press the points listed in the entries for Anxiety, page 42, and Stress, page 95, to relax.

Replace the fluids lost through sweating with clear liquids such as water or chilled herbal teas. Drinking at least one glass an hour helps you feel cooler. Peppermint and spearmint teas can be made in quantity and refrigerated. Echinacea tea is an herbal antibiotic and temperature stabilizer. Steep one teaspoon of the dried herb in one cup of boiling water until cool enough to drink.

Flatulence

Flatulence is a tiresome and embarrassing problem associated with digestive dysfunction, overeating, and nervousness (see the entry for Stress, page 95). An excess of spicy foods, sugar, or fats can cause several kinds of digestive disturbance. Some people find that flatulence disappears when they limit their fruit intake to two or three pieces per day.

Eastern health practitioners treat flatulence as a symptom of imbalance in the Earth and Metal meridians. These regulate digestion and elimination. In addition to suggesting possible dietary changes, they treat Large Intestine 1 and 9, Spleen 3, and Stomach 45.

Also see the entry for Stomach/Abdominal Discomfort, page 94.

Foot Pain

Foot pain can result from an injury, unsuitable footwear, or poor postural habits (particularly during repeated motions). When your feet hurt, look for the cause instead of attempting to ignore the pain—this will help you avoid disabling injury. Check for obvious problems like bruises or muscle strain, which you can treat with acupressure. Press Golden Points to relieve muscle fatigue and improve circulation; you can make this part of your warm-up and cool-down routines.

If your pain persists, evaluate your footwear. Are you wearing the proper shoes for your sport? For example, a shoe designed for aerobic dancing or racquet sports will not absorb the slamming shock your feet receive during a run or race-walk. Purchase your shoes from a knowledgeable salesperson who asks specific questions about your exercise participation and goals. Runners and walkers must have adequate heel support, since your heel takes the full impact of your weight during large muscle exercise.

Recurrent heel pain could indicate heel spurs, which can be protected with heel pads that are available in drugstores. You can also improvise your own with moleskin taped over your heels before exercising.

If your foot pain persists despite self-treatment, consult a podiatrist or sports physician. These doctors can order X rays and other tests to identify structural problems.

Foreskin Irritation

See Balanitis, page 45.

Gout

Gout is a form of arthritis that manifests as painful swelling in one or both big toes. This makes movement difficult. It is typically aggravated by heavy or tight-fitting footwear that restricts circulation.

Relieve gout pain with acupressure, warm-water soaks, and comfortable footwear. Soak your foot in a pan of warm water for fifteen minutes. Then press Spleen 1 (not to be used in pregnancy), Spleen 3, Liver 1, Liver 2, Liver 3, and Stomach 42. This can be done several times a day to relieve pain and stiffness. When your symptoms resolve, continue pressing these points once daily to prevent a recurrence.

Evaluate your footwear (see the entry for Foot Pain, page 68). Tight shoes with pointed toes inhibit circulation and aggravate swollen, painful feet. Wear comfortable slippers or sandals whenever possible (these can be worn with socks in cold weather).

Hay Fever

Hay fever is a collection of symptoms that includes swollen nasal membranes; the pressure from these results in frontal headache and labored breathing. Hay fever can also give you a runny nose and red, itchy eyes. It typically appears in the form of an allergic response to blooming plants, and symptoms may also be triggered by household chemicals, industrial pollutants, or a host of other allergens. Macrobiotic health practitioners feel that dairy products increase mucus within the body, thus aggravating sinus discomfort.

Acupressure relieves stuffed sinuses, easing pressure and pain. Start your treatment by pressing Bladder 2 on both sides of your face. Apply a gradual upward pressure with your index finger (this is easiest when you lie on your back). Maintain the pressure for at least five minutes to obtain the maximum relief. Continue your acupressure treatment with Triple Warmer 23, then Stomach 3, concluding with Governing Vessel 26. If your eyes itch and tear, add Bladder 1, Gall Bladder 1, and Gall Bladder 14. You can also press Spleen 7 to relieve the itching.

Conclude your sinus treatment by pressing Liver 1 and 3. This strengthens the Liver meridian, which plays an important role in filtering allergens from your body.

Headache

Head pain has many causes, including stress response, sinus congestion, or exposure to allergens. Temporomandibular Joint Syndrome can also cause headache (see the entry for Bruxism, page 50). Headache usually begins with muscular tension. This causes blood vessel spasms in upper body muscles, reducing blood flow. The muscles signal to the brain that they have a smaller blood volume, and the brain responds with pain.

Most people attempt to treat headaches with over the counter remedies such as aspirin or Tylenol. However, severe and recurrent pain should be treated by a neurologist. For minor, relatively infrequent head pain, acupressure can be a safe alternative remedy. Acupressure relaxes tense muscles, thus interrupting the pain producing cycle. Begin treatment with a few deep relaxed breaths, then gently massage your entire scalp to break up stiffness. Press in with your fingertips, moving the entire hand and wrist in a circular motion. When you have rubbed your entire scalp, choose points near the pain center.

For *frontal headache*, press Bladder 2, Gall Bladder 1 and 14, Triple Warmer 23, Governing Vessel 4, and Stomach 6 (also see the entry for Hay Fever, page 69).

For *occipital headache* (back of the head), press Triple Warmer 16 and 19, Gall Bladder 19 and 20, and Governing Vessel 17.

For *pain on the top of the head*, press Gall Bladder 15, 16, 17, 18, Bladder 5 and 8, and Governing Vessel 20 and 22.

For *pain on the sides of the head*, press Triple Warmer 23, Small Intestine 19, Gall Bladder 4 and 20, and Stomach 6 and 7.

Complete your treatment with points to relax your neck and shoulders (see the entry for Joint Pain and Stiffness, page 78).

Heartburn

Heartburn is a fiery sensation in your throat or chest, typically occurring during a meal or immediately afterward. You are most vulnerable to heartburn when you have eaten too quickly or have consumed more food than your stomach can comfortably hold. Pregnant women occasionally suffer from heartburn after the first trimester, when an enlarged uterus compresses the stomach.

For quick relief, press Stomach 42 and Spleen 4, which balance the Earth element. Pregnant acupressure clients also find it beneficial to eat small amounts of food every two to three hours for the duration of a pregnancy. Research suggests that tobacco, coffee, and chocolate interfere with the digestive process in a manner that intensifies heartburn.

Hemorrhoids

Hemorrhoids are widened veins that appear as small purple growths of skin around the anus. A colonic examination may also show these itchy painful growths inside the rectum. Hemorrhoids sometimes appear during pregnancy, when added weight in the lower abdomen slows lower body circulation. Constipation may also have this effect (see the entry for Constipation, page 57).

For relief, sit in a warm bath for at least half an hour every day. Press acupressure points to relieve the itching and promote healthy circulation and bowel function. Spleen 7 is the traditional remedy for itching, while Governing Vessel 2 and Large Intestine 1 and 4 (not to be used in pregnancy) promote healthy bowels.

You can also use a potato suppository to soothe pain and itching. Carve a piece of unpeeled potato to the size of your little finger. The edges should be rounded. Insert this suppository into the anus and replace it every four to six hours.

Hernia

Hernia is a weakness or opening in a wall of muscle or connective tissue. An organ may protrude through it. Hernias are usually a male health problem, and an *inguinal hernia* is the most common type. This appears in the groin and probably extends to the scrotum. Another type is the *hiatal hernia*, which afflicts the diaphragm, the muscle separating the abdominal and chest cavities. With hiatal hernia, eating can be difficult. Stomach acid flows backward from the stomach into the esophagus, which causes a heartburnlike irritation (see the entry for Heartburn, page 71). Other types are *incisional hernias* that develop at the site of previous surgery, and *umbilical hernias*, weaknesses in the muscle wall or connective tissue surrounding the navel. Some infants are born with umbilical hernias. These generally heal by the time the children are four, and surgical intervention is rarely prescribed.

If your doctor says you have a hernia, she will probably advise you to avoid heavy lifting, and to discuss any new exercise program with her. In addition, you can probably control mild hernia discomfort naturally. Increase healthy circulation around your hernia by pressing the nearby Golden Points. (Pressing directly into the affected area may cause further pain.) Classical acupressure points for hernia treatment are Gall Bladder 14, 30, 40, and 41; Liver 1, 3, and 14; Bladder 27, 28, 47; and Governing Vessel 2 and 4. Press at least three of these points every day to increase circulation and muscle flexibility. If you have pain, rest while you press the rest of the points. Hot and cold compresses provide further relief. Place a hot compress against the painful area. Let it remain for five minutes, then immediately replace it with an ice pack, which also remains on for five minutes. Continue until your pain is relieved. If your pain continues, however, you must consult your doctor.

A hernia is not considered a medical emergency unless it becomes *incarcerated*, that is, it cannot be pressed down without severe pain, and you feel a swollen, tender mass. Your bowel movements stop if this mass blocks your intestines. Your abdomen is probably distended, and you are nauseated and have uncontrollable vomiting. If you have these symptoms, you require emergency medical care.

Herpes

Herpes is a viral infection. Its most obvious symptoms are small, round, itchy blisters on the skin. These are most often seen around your mouth (Simplex 1) and genitals (Simplex 2). The blisters can break open, become runny, and scab over, particularly when the outbreak has nearly run its course. At this time, your lymph nodes may also be swollen. Flulike fatigue and weakness also characterize herpes. You are most vulnerable to an outbreak when you are tired, tense, or ill.

To relieve the itching, press Spleen 7 as often as necessary. You can also use goldenseal or green-clay poultices. Mix one of these substances with a little water, pack it on the blisters, and let it dry. (Wash your hands immediately after application!) Keep your genital area clean with glycerine soap and water, and wash any clothing that touches your genitals, including swimsuits and leotards, each time you wear them. Be sure that these clothes are especially well rinsed, as laundry detergent can be irritating; add minimal soap when you do your wash, and do a second hand rinse before it goes in the dryer.

Do not attempt to self-diagnose herpes. The blisters could indicate another venereal disease or an allergy. Consult a physician for testing and diagnosis. Herpes is extremely infectious, so refrain from any sexual contact (including kissing and oral sex) when sores are present. If you accidentally touch the sores, wash your hands immediately.

Hives

Hives are swollen, itchy patches on the skin that often appear in response to stress, insect bites, or some foods and medicines.

They sometimes develop in the throat mucosal tissue, causing difficulty in breathing and swallowing. If you suffer from hives you may be allergic to dairy products, shellfish, chocolate, or strawberries. Be sure to call your doctor if hives appear while you're taking antibiotics or some other prescribed medication. (See the entry for Contact Dermatitis, page 58.)

Press Spleen 7 to relieve the itching, and then press Large Intestine 1 and Lung 9 to tone the Metal meridians that govern skin health. For hives in your throat, simultaneously press Conception Vessel 21 and 24.

You can also use a goldenseal poultice to reduce the itching and swelling. (Goldenseal should not be used in pregnancy.) Grind the dried herb in a mortar and pestle (or buy it in powdered form if available). Mix the ground herb with a little warm water—just enough to make a paste that is directly applied to the hives. Let the paste dry before you rinse it off. For best results, relax and press acupressure points while it's drying.

You may also be interested in acupressure stress reduction, since relaxation training has been helpful to some clients with hives. (See the entries for Anxiety, page 42, and Stress, page 95.)

Impotence

Impotence is a man's inability to achieve or sustain an erection, making some kinds of sexual activity impossible. Nearly all men are impotent at some time. This is usually distressing, since the problem is commonly associated with age and infirmity. While erections do become less frequent as a man ages, there are other possible causes. Stress, lack of confidence, and relationship problems have all been implicated in short-term impotence. (Your body may be telling you that sexual contact is inappropriate at this point in your connection with a lover.) Some prescription drugs temporarily interfere with sexual functioning. If your impotence dates from the first day you took a medication, don't be embarrassed to discuss the problem with your doctor. He can probably supply an alternate prescription.

Continuing or chronic impotence usually has a physiological cause. For example, diabetic men sometimes have difficulty in getting an erection. Fortunately, even chronic impotence is today often treatable and curable. Consult a urologist if the problem does not resolve itself within a few weeks.

In Asian medicine sexual dysfunction is associated with the Fire and Water meridians. Working with acupressure clients has taught me that sexual dysfunction originating from physical disease is usually a Water problem. If the cause is emotion centered, it will be most effectively treated with Fire.

Asian physicians regard sexual dysfunction as a symptom of low energy in the Water meridians. In addition to using acupressure for instant relief during the acute stage, press at least one of these points daily: Kidney 1, Kidney 3, Kidney 7, Kidney 11, Conception Vessel 2, Governing Vessel 14, Heart 7 and 9, Pericardium 8, and Triple Warmer 1.

Influenza (Flu)

Flu is often mistaken for the common cold. While colds affect the upper respiratory system, flu also involves the bronchial tubes and the lungs. The first symptoms of influenza are aching muscles, exhaustion, and a general "I can't cope" feeling. Nausea, vomiting, and fever may follow. The fever is higher than that with a cold. These symptoms typically last from one to seven days. When you have the flu, your respiratory system is vulnerable to harmful bacteria. Untreated flu can lead to other diseases like strep throat and ear infections. Flu is very contagious and usually occurs in epidemics. You must avoid infecting other people, particularly young children, frail elderly people, pregnant or nursing women, and the chronically ill, since they are all particularly vulnerable.

You can make yourself less vulnerable to flu viruses by getting enough rest and following good nutritional habits. Stress, over-work, and an inadequate diet often precede viral illnesses. Supplement your regular diet with a multivitamin supplement during cold weather or stressful periods.

If you get the flu, rest in bed until your symptoms subside, and use acupressure and herbs to make you more comfortable. Refer to the entries for Fever (page 66), Stomach/Abdominal Discomfort (page 94), and Stress (page 95).

Injection Pain

Minimize the sting of a "shot" by preparing a hot comfrey poultice before the injection. Cut a clean piece of unbleached muslin into a piece about the size of your hand. Put two table-spoons of dried comfrey in the center of the cloth, and fold the edges over the herb. Then pour hot water from a teakettle over the covered herb. Apply the poultice to the injection site when the needle is removed.

While the poultice cools on your skin, press Golden Points near the injection site to increase circulation.

Insect Stings

Insect stings cause brief pain and upset to most adults and children. When you are stung, rinse the insect's target area with cool water, and apply ice to numb the sting. Press the ice against the sting for at least ten minutes while you relax. (See A Calming Meditation on page 43.) You can also press Liver 1 and 3, traditionally used to help your body release unhealthy substances.

Be alert to unusual responses to the sting. If you are suscepti-ble to bee venom and other insect-secreted substances, your body recognizes a threat. Its responses include swelling and a rash that may appear anywhere on your body; choking and breathing difficulties; nausea and stomach/abdominal discomfort; and fainting. You may lose consciousness abruptly. Any of these symptoms may indicate anaphylactic shock syndrome. This severe allergic response causes sudden, severe blood vessel constriction in the entire body; shock, cardiac arrest, and even death can result without immediate care at a doctor's office or emergency room.

If you are vulnerable to anaphylactic shock syndrome, you must always have a predetermined plan for getting the medical care you need if stung.

Also see the entries for Anxiety, page 42, and Shock, page 92.

Insomnia

Insomnia, the inability to sleep, is a common symptom of stress. It also results from overexcitement, consuming too much sugar and coffee after dinner, or trying to sleep before you are calm and relaxed. Bladder problems are another cause of sleeplessness. It's difficult to get a full night's rest when you have to keep going to the toilet. (See the entry for Urinary Incontinence, page 98.) Children often cannot sleep if they are peremptorily ordered to bed, or forbidden to read or listen to quiet music before an arbitrary lights-out time. A nightly hour of predictable, relaxed activity before bedtime usually calms both adults and children enough to sleep.

Over the counter drugs and alcohol ostensibly relax you and put an end to insomniac frustration. However, these may actually suppress your capacity for restful, dreaming sleep. Replace these Western tranquilizers with concentrated acupressure practice. Press Heart 7, Heart 9, Kidney 3, Kidney 8, and Lung 1.

Jock Rot

Jock rot is the common name for a hot, itchy skin irritation that typically occurs on the upper legs near the genitals. It may be caused by a fungus, or by the friction of clothing against the skin.

Heat intensifies your symptoms. You are most susceptible to jock rot during lengthy workouts when you perspire heavily.

To treat jock rot, see Contact Dermatitis, page 58.

Joint Pain and Stiffness

Joint pain and stiffness limit your activity and sense of well-being. While frequent discomfort can be a symptom of arthritis or other disease, much joint pain is caused and aggravated by poor body mechanics, lack of exercise, or some other correctable problem. You can improve your posture by cultivating an awareness of the way you sit, stand, and move. (See A Walking Meditation on page 81.) For example, minimize upper body stiffness and fatigue by alternating loads from side to side. If you routinely carry heavy objects (such as a briefcase, or a young child), hold them with your left hand or arm for a few minutes, then change sides.

If your exercise program consists mainly of large muscle activity such as running or jogging, joint pain is probably your body's way of saying enough. Dr. Stan James, an orthopedist who treats Olympic runners, claims that two-thirds of all running injuries are caused by overly ambitious and rigid training programs. He recommends that workout duration and intensity increase gradually, supplemented by rest days and alternative forms of exercise. Swimming is an alternative large muscle activity that stretches and tones muscles while providing an aerobic workout. A yoga class will teach you relaxing postures to counteract muscle strain from high-impact exercise such as tennis or running. Iyengar yoga emphasizes correct postural alignment to bring your attention to pain-producing habits. (To find a yoga class that's right for you, see Resources, page 131.) Sheila, a marathon runner, switched to cross-training (which combines exercise activities) when her knees began to bother her. She investigated local gymnasium facilities, finally settling on a facility that offered supervised weight lifting and a pool. After several months of these alternative workouts, Sheila found that she could still run twice a week without stressing her knees.

Acupressure is therapeutic, relaxing tight, tense muscles. You can press points in a problem area each day. For example, if you are prone to hip pain, you can press the points listed below each morning or evening. You can also make acupressure a part of your exercise routine. Press points before and after your workout to increase flexibility.

For hip tension, press Gall Bladder 30 and 31, Bladder 47, 48, 49, and 50, Governing Vessel 2 and 4, and Spleen 12. For shoulder stiffness, press Large Intestine 14 and 15, Small Intestine 11, Bladder 38, Gall Bladder 21, and Governing Vessel 13 and 15. For leg tightness, see entries for Cramps, page 58, Foot Pain, page 68, Shin Splints, page 91, and Knee Injury, page 79.

Knee Injury

Knee injuries can range from simple (although painful) sprains to more serious damage, such as the severing of knee ligaments. Robert Johnson, M.D., an orthopedics rehabilitation specialist at the University of Vermont, claims that knee injuries are the most commonly diagnosed ski injury. They nearly always limit your activity. Knee trauma often needs extra time and attention to heal, since the knees bear much of your weight and are constantly bending and straightening.

When you hurt your knee, *stop what you're doing at once!* If the pain is intense, or lasts longer than a minute or two, do not resume the activity. Apply the classic RICE technique (rest, ice, compression, elevation) as soon as possible, and press Bladder 54 to relieve muscular tension and promote circulation.

To apply RICE, lie on a bed or sofa or sit in a chair with a comfortable footrest. Slide a thick pillow under your injured knee, and prop an ice pack directly over the injury while you read, do needlework, watch television, and so on. Every half hour, lean forward and press Bladder 54, located in the center of the crease at the back of your knee, for five minutes at a time. (A relaxed muscle feels better than a tense tight one!) Supplement RICE and Bladder 54 with Bladder 38, Kidney 3, and Stomach 36.

Several of my acupressure clients found RICE most helpful during the first forty-eight hours after the injury. Thereafter, a system of alternating hot and cold compresses gave more effective pain relief. Begin this treatment by applying a hot, wet washcloth (don't burn yourself!) to the injured area, and let it remain there for five minutes. Then replace it with an ice pack that also stays on for five minutes. Repeat as often as necessary to relieve the pain.

PREVENTING SPORTS INJURY

- *Begin any exercise with slow stretching and gradually build up intensity.*
- *If you work out first thing in the morning, increase warm-up time. Your joints and muscles are generally stiffest (and most prone to injury) during the first two hours of your day.*
- *When taking up a new sport, be certain that you have the proper equipment—if you rent or borrow it, make sure that everything fits you properly.*
- *Hire a professional instructor or trainer who will teach you the correct body mechanics for your sport. (Also see the walking meditation that follows. Practiced regularly, this exercise will teach you to evaluate the way in which you move and carry yourself.)*
- *Break in new shoes by wearing them for an hour or two each day until they feel comfortable.*

Laryngitis

Laryngitis is a viral or bacterial infection of the larynx (voice box). It usually follows a respiratory tract infection (such as a cold) and produces hoarseness and a sore throat. (See the entry for Pharyngitis, page 87.)

Fluids relieve laryngitis throat discomfort. Drink several cups of boneset tea every day. This herb, a classic remedy for the respiratory tract, is purchased dry at a health food store or herbal supply shop. (See Resources, page 131.) Steep one teaspoon of boneset in a cup of boiling water until it is cool enough to drink. Mint teas like spearmint and peppermint are also soothing and pleasant tasting.

A WALKING MEDITATION

This meditation alerts you to postural habits that contribute to discomfort and injury.

Take off your shoes, and make sure that the floor in front of you is free of potential hazards such as toys, pins, and so on.

Close your eyes. Take several deep breaths. Step forward, and observe your physical sensations. What parts of your foot are touching the ground? Take another step. How much weight do you put on your heels? On the balls of your feet? Do your knees feel flexible, or do you suddenly become aware that you habitually keep them stiff? What do your ankles feel like?

Notice how the ground beneath you supports your weight and keeps you in balance. You were constructed to live and move naturally on the earth. Let yourself relax into the support of gravity; you don't need to hold yourself up.

What are you doing with your arms and shoulders as you walk? You don't need to hold them up either. Keep walking (open your eyes if you need to!), and keep observing.

Stimulate a soothing flow of saliva by simultaneously pressing Conception Vessel 21 and 24. Be sure to presss for at least five minutes at a time for the maximum relief.

Rest as much as possible. Try not to talk, don't eat scratchy foods (crackers, potato chips, French bread), and *don't smoke*.

Take care of other respiratory problems, such as a cold or tonsillitis. (See the entries for Colds and Bronchitis, page 54, and Pharyngitis, page 87.)

Liver Pain

Liver pain occurs on your right side, next to your elbow. Typically it is a short, sharp pain that feels like a knife slice. You may notice it when you overeat or take chemical medication.

Press Liver 1, 3, and 14 for pain relief. For further relief, relax with a hot gingerroot compress over your liver. Severe or recurrent pain may signify a serious problem and it must be brought to your doctor's attention.

The liver separates usable food and drug substances from those the body must discard. When this important organ is overworked, pain can result. During periods of liver stress, you can press liver-strengthening acupressure points. For example, you can press points when taking prescription medication, or while overeating during holidays or a vacation. Liver 1, 3, and 14, Gall Bladder 40, and Kidney 7 (not to be used in pregnancy) are good liver strengtheners.

Asian herbalists prescribe sour mugwort tea for their patients with liver pain. Mugwort, a vegetable, is found in the produce section of Asian groceries and in some health food stores. Chop one tablespoon of the peeled mugwort, and steep it in boiling water until it is cool enough to drink. You may drink up to two cups a day. Children under fifteen take half this dose.

Menstrual Cramps

Menstrual cramps, or period pain, range from mild discomfort to intense, disabling pain. Since these cramps are actually uterine muscle spasms, self-treatment begins with relaxation. (See the entries for Stress, page 95, and Anxiety, page 42.) Press Spleen 3, 4, 6 (not to be used in pregnancy), 10, and 12; Conception Vessel 2 and 4; and Stomach 36 and 42 to relieve menstrual cramps. If you suffer from period pain each month, you may find it helpful to press at least three of these points each day for one week before menstruation is expected.

Supplement your acupressure points with herbal and nutritional remedies for severe cramping. Valerian tea is a strong, natural muscle relaxant. Steep one teaspoonful of the dried herb in a cup of boiling hot water until it is cool enough to drink.

Alternatively, take one thousand milligrams of calcium and magnesium (sometimes marketed as dolomite) with some heated milk. Do not use either of these relaxation inducing remedies before driving.

Monilia (Yeast Infection)

Monilia, popularly known as yeast infection, is characterized by genital itching, burning, and discharge. (A doctor can test you to find out if you really have monilia or some other form of vaginitis, such as trichomonas.) You are subject to monilia if the Lactobacillus flora, which helps keep the genital pH sufficiently acidic, is disrupted, making you vulnerable to yeast. The Lactobacillus flora can be disrupted by hormonal changes, a sudden depletion of B vitamins, or drugs. Antibiotics and birth-control pills have been identified as yeast-causing culprits, along with chemical bath products, lubricants, and spermicides. Some of these can be eliminated or replaced with other products. (See Resources, page 131.)

Relieve itching by pressing Spleen 7 and Kidney 11. Press each point for at least five minutes. You can also get quick relief by swallowing several acidophilus tablets (if your health food store doesn't carry these, see Resources, page 131).

If your yeast problem persists, use acupressure and dietary aids to create genital health. Acupressure relaxation enables you to release tension and get enough rest, thus balancing acidity levels. (See the entries for Anxiety, page 42, Fatigue, page 65, and Stress, page 95.) There are also specific points that benefit the urogenital organs. Press three of these points daily for one month after your yeast symptoms resolve: Kidney 1, Kidney 3, Kidney 7, Kidney 11, Bladder 64, and Conception Vessel 2. This will help prevent a recurrence. If you need antibiotics or birth-control pills, you may prevent a yeast problem before it begins by pressing points and taking acidophilus capsules on the day that you begin medication.

Cleanliness is essential if you want to rid yourself of a yeast infection. You probably change your underwear every day, but remember that other clothing that touches the genitals (leotards, swimsuits) must be washed before you wear it again. Use your own towel and washcloth so you don't spread the yeast infection to anyone else.

Nasal Congestion

Nasal and sinus congestion can result from colds, bronchitis, or responses to allergens such as pollens or air pollution. Congestion makes breathing hard work, a tiring and irritating problem.

To relieve congestion, press Bladder 2, Stomach 6, and Triple Warmer 23. Also see the entries for Asthma, page 44, Breathing Difficulties, page 49, Colds and Bronchitis, page 54, Croup, page 110, and Hay Fever, page 69.

Nausea

Nausea can have numerous causes. Your stomach can become queasy in response to overeating, motion, emotional upset (see the entry for Anxiety, page 42), or as a result of the onset of an illness such as influenza (see the entry for Influenza, page 75). It can also be a side effect of some foods and medications, if you are sensitive to these substances. (If you are taking a prescription medication, be sure to notify your doctor if you experience this unpleasant side effect.)

Press Spleen 3 and Stomach 42 for prompt relief of nausea, since the Earth meridians regulate the digestive organs. Most foods will increase your nausea. However, chewing a few dry crackers slowly and thoroughly sometimes relieves mild queasiness. Mint teas are another traditional tonic. Steep one teaspoon of spearmint or peppermint tea in one cup of boiling water until the tea is cool enough to drink, and then sip it slowly. (The cooled tea can also be put in a baby's bottle.) Mint teas may be drunk freely.

Also see the entry for Vomiting, page 100.

Panic

Panic disorders are common in Western society. The Phobia Society of America estimates that 4 to 8 percent of the American public suffers from periodic bouts of dizziness, intense fear, and pounding heart brought on by an unwelcome rush of adrenaline. Panic attacks also include perspiring, tingling palms, and vertigo. Most sufferers do not seek medical assistance, preferring to endure these troubling symptoms rather than make them known to others.

Dr. Richard A. Lannon of the Langley-Porter Neuropsychiatric Institute believes that panic attacks begin in a section of the brain called the locus ceruleus, which secretes adrenaline and other hormones. Rushes of fear-stimulating hormones in the locus ceruleus may bring on symptoms. Dr. Lannon states that sedatives apparently do not help this condition.

Acupressure clients with panic and anxiety disorders were helped by stress reduction. They used acupressure and meditation techniques (see the entry for Anxiety, page 42) to slow breathing, calm pounding hearts, and restore emotional equilibrium. Focusing attention on self-help rather than on troublesome symptoms brought positive results.

Pelvic Pain

Pelvic pain in women results from tension, sexual problems, or physical disease, including endometriosis, pelvic inflammatory disease (PID), and bladder infections. If you use a birth control device such as a diaphragm, it may not have been inserted properly or carefully fit upon prescription.

Intercourse is sometimes painful when a woman is not sufficiently aroused before her vagina is penetrated. A caring partner will be eager to make sex comfortable and enjoyable if you communicate your need for more foreplay. Insufficient vaginal lubrication is a problem for many women in their fifties, when a drop in estrogen affects lubricity. Asian medical practitioners associate vaginal dryness with the kidneys, a center of sexual and reproductive energy. They treat Kidney 1, Kidney 3, and Conception Vessel 2. These points are pressed daily for a recurring problem, or they may be incorporated into sexual foreplay.

Pelvic stiffness and pain during lovemaking has other causes. If you are tense and tight all over, you may find it difficult to enjoy lovemaking and even receive your lover without pain. Take time to relax with your partner before you initiate sex. Listen to music, talk quietly, and press Acupressure points on each other's bodies. Press Governing Vessel 2 and 4, Gall Bladder 30, and Bladder 42 and 47 to relax your pelvic area.

Relationship problems can also lead to sexual dysfunction. If you feel unresolved anger or disappointment, sometimes you literally can't take your lover. For example, young women may suffer from such intense tightening of the vaginal muscles (gynecologists call this vaginismus) that intercourse is difficult or impossible. If you feel pressured, anxious, or resentful, this may be your body's conscientious objection to the sexual act.

Your pelvic tension may also be residue from a traumatic sexual experience. Women who have been raped sometimes have difficulty in separating this act of violence from sexual union with a loving partner. A period of celibacy is a helpful coping mechanism, along with counseling from an experienced and sensitive psychological services professional.

Pelvic pain is sometimes psychogenic (originating in your emotions), but recurrent discomfort should be checked out by your doctor. She can examine you and order tests to determine whether you have a gynecological disease.

Also see Bladder Symptoms, page 46.

Penis Irritation

See Balanitis, page 45, Bladder Symptoms, page 46, Epididymitis, page 63, Prostate Symptoms, page 90, and Testicle Torsion, page 96.

Pharyngitis (Sore Throat)

A sore throat usually accompanies a cold or some other upper respiratory tract infection. Your throat becomes dry, scratchy, and red. Exposure to tear gas, tobacco, and marijuana also can cause a sore throat if you're susceptible. A dry indoor environment (like most living spaces in the winter) can aggravate a sore throat, so consider using a humidifier. When you have a sore throat, you may be hoarse for about half a day, with sore and swollen lymph nodes. Check with your doctor if you have a high fever, chills, or muscular aches, as these are signs of strep throat and require your doctor's attention.

Nurse a sore throat with plenty of rest, liquids, and acupressure. Relax in bed and drink a cup of water or herbal tea every hour to soothe your throat. Comfrey tea is an excellent tonic. Use one teaspoon of the dried herb to one cup of boiling water. Steep it until it is cool enough to drink. Conception Vessel 21 and 24 relax your throat and stimulate a soothing flow of saliva. Press these points simultaneously until you feel relief. (This requires you to press for five to ten minutes.)

If your doctor says you have strep throat, use these points to supplement her prescribed treatment.

Poison Exposure or Ingestion

If you accidentally consume or become exposed to a poisonous substance, immediately call your local poison control center, doctor's office, or local emergency telephone service for advice. Describe the poison, reading the label to the emergency worker if necessary, and follow their instructions to the letter.

While you're waiting for emergency help, remember the following:

- If you've been exposed to poisonous vapors, get out into the open air;
- If a dangerous substance lands on your skin, flush the exposed area with copious amounts of clear water; do not induce vomiting if gasoline or kerosene have been ingested, as this may further damage the nose and throat.

Reduce the chance of poison ingestion by careful storage of all substances such as cleaners, paint, or automotive fluids. If you have hazardous materials in your home, garage, or workplace, you should understand how to store and use them safely. Any potential hazards must be kept out of the reach of children and pets. For assistance with this, contact your local poison control center or Red Cross office. Press Heart 7 and 9, Pericardium 5, Stomach 42, and Spleen 3 to relax and calm the poisoning victim while you wait for emergency help; you can also press Liver

3 and Large Intestine 1 and 4 (not used in pregnancy) to strengthen the body's resistance to toxins.

Poison Oak, Ivy, or Sumac

The Girl Scouts say it best: "Leaves of three, let it be!" Many people are sensitive to poison oak, ivy, or sumac, which are distinguished by their threefold leaf structure. If one of these plants has touched your skin, immediately wash it with soap and water and rinse repeatedly. Then wash your hands and fingernails (they retain volatile oils from the leaves). Washing can prevent or minimize symptom onset, or can minimize severity.

About eight hours after you touch the plant, a raised, bright red area will appear on your skin. This is dotted with small pimples, some containing water or pus. This rash is extremely itchy but must not be scratched. Scratching breaks the pimples, spreading the pus and, consequently, the rash. Your symptoms will normally resolve within seven to ten days if you can keep yourself from scratching.

You can use acupressure and herbal remedies to soothe the itching and stimulate healing circulation to your infected skin. Press Spleen 7 as often as you feel the itching. For the maximum relief, press steadily for at least five to ten minutes at a time. You can also press Large Intestine 1, 4 (not to be used in pregnancy), and 11, and Lung 9, associated with skin health. David found that a paste of powdered goldenseal herb relieved his itching. He applied the paste three times a day until the rash faded. David pressed points before going to sleep at night to minimize scratching during the night.

Moderate amounts of water and light may also speed recovery. Jennifer worried that the poison oak that covered much of her skin surface would disrupt a Carribean vacation. Instead, the sunlight and seawater apparently dried up the rash, speeding her recovery.

When you apply sunscreen or herbal paste, or touch the rash for any reason, wash your hands immediately to avoid spreading your symptoms.

Also see Chapped Skin, page 52, Contact Dermatitis, page 58, Hives, page 73, and Psoriasis, page 90.

Prostate Symptoms

The prostate gland produces the fluid that combines with the secretion from the testes to form a man's ejaculate. It is located below the bladder, close to the urethra. A swollen prostate presses against the urethra, blocking the urine flow. After several days of this urine retention, you may feel slightly achy and tired. You are also susceptible to urethral and bladder infections. Treat the discomfort of an enlarged prostate with acupressure and warm gingerroot compresses. Press Conception Vessel 3 and Spleen 6. To make the compress, peel and chop about a tablespoonful of fresh gingerroot (available in groceries and health food stores), wrap it in a clean square of unbleached muslin, and pour hot water over it. When this compress is cool enough to handle, set it over your bladder. You may also find it soothing to make a larger gingerroot compress and place it over your kidneys.

Press Kidney 1 and 3, Bladder 64, and Conception Vessel 6 twice each day until your symptoms disappear. Then continue pressing these points daily for two weeks thereafter to help prevent recurrence.

Psoriasis

Psoriasis is a skin disease that manifests in bright red patches covered with silvery scales. The patches are painful, especially when touched, and they sometimes itch. They can clear up in a few days or weeks, but chronic psoriasis is not rare.

Psoriasis should be washed and dried thoroughly at least twice a day. Stimulate healthy circulation to the surface skin layers by pressing nearby Golden Points, and supplement these with green-clay poultices.

If your psoriasis is itchy, press Spleen 7 as needed for relief. Asian health practitioners supplement this symptomatic treatment with Metal meridian points, since this element governs skin health. If you suffer from psoriasis or other skin problems on a regular basis, press at least two of these points each day: Large Intestine 1, 4 (not to be used in pregnancy), 5, and 20; Lung 2, 7 (not to be used in pregnancy), and 9.

You can also soothe dry, irritated skin with applications of aloe vera gel or jojoba oil (see Resources, page 131). Fish oil, a staple in health food stores, proved beneficial in one study on twenty-eight patients with chronic psoriasis. Half of the group took ten capsules of fish oil each day, while the remainder swallowed placebos. The patients who received the placebo had no change in symptoms, but all members of the treatment group reported significant decreases in itching and scaling.

Also see the entries for Chapped Skin, page 52, and Contact Dermatitis, page 58.

Rash

See Contact Dermatitis, page 58.

Scrotum Inflammation and Infection

See Epididymitis, page 63, Prostate Symptoms, page 90, and Testicle Torsion, page 97.

Shin Splints

"Shin splint" is the term most used to describe pain and stiffness in the lower legs. The medical definition includes swelling and mild to moderate muscle tearing, and the pain intensifies when you walk or run. In severe cases, the muscle is stiff and sensitive to the touch. Direct finger pressure on points will probably be too painful, so begin your self-treatment with RICE (see page 79) and massage.

Rub a natural oil, such as safflower or peanut oil, into your hands. Then rub your palms over your calves in wide, circular motions. Be sure to rub the hamstring muscle that runs up the back of your leg. Press in lightly without forcing or pinching. As your muscles loosen up, you can increase the palm pressure. Rub each leg for at least three minutes two (or more) times each day for relief.

If your muscles are softened enough for finger pressure, press at least three of these points: Bladder 54, 58, and 60; Kidney 3; Liver 3 and 5; Stomach 36 and 42; and Gall Bladder 40, 41, and 44. Consult the charts on pages 26–27 and 32–33 to determine which points are nearest your leg pain.

If you find that pressing points near the pain site is too painful, you can always use other points that aren't so close. You will still benefit from the increased circulation and muscular tension release.

Shock

Shock is your body's response to physical or psychological trauma. Its symptoms include cold hands, pale facial skin, and dizziness or fainting. If you have an injury, pain may be minimal or absent. The most common shock symptom, however, is mental disorientation. Shock keeps you from responding appropriately to the situation at hand. For example, you may refuse medical treatment despite an obvious injury.

Preschool children, pregnant women, and the elderly are particularly susceptible to shock and should be carefully watched for symptoms following an accident or other trauma.

Shock is a medical emergency regardless of other injury. Blood vessels constrict, reducing the circulation that carries sustaining oxygen to vital cells. You can help a shock patient waiting for emergency care by having him lie down with his feet elevated. Press calming acupressure points that will relax his breathing. Kidney 1 (not to be used in pregnancy), Lung 1 and 2, Heart 7 and 9, Pericardium 5, and Conception Vessel 17 are good points for shock patients. Use a particularly slow and gentle touch.

Shoulder Stiffness

See Joint Pain and Stiffness, page 78.

Smoke Inhalation

The first step in treating smoke inhalation is to move away from the smoky area. Get to fresh air as quickly as possible. Heat, smoke, and chemical fumes can cause severe damage to your respiratory system.

Early signs of heat and smoke injury include hoarseness, coughing, and difficulty in swallowing. Prolonged inhalation can cause mucosa in the lungs to swell and shatter, leaking fluid that plugs the air passages. This causes severe oxygen reduction, a condition that leads to suffocation if it is not promptly treated by emergency medical workers.

To relieve congestion in the early stages of heat and smoke inhalation, press Bladder 2, Stomach 6, and Triple Warmer 23. Press Conception Vessel 21 and 24 to relieve hoarseness and sore throat. See a doctor promptly if your symptoms last more than half an hour.

Also see the entries for Asthma, page 44, Breathing Diffi-culties, page 49, Colds and Bronchitis, page 54, Croup, page 110, Hay Fever, page 69, and Pharyngitis, page 87.

Sore Throat

See Pharyngitis, page 87.

Stitch in the Side

"I've got a stitch in my side," is the common explanation for a sudden sharp pain in the upper right side of the abdomen. Your doctor calls this round ligament spasm. It is common in the third trimester of pregnancy and during strenuous exercise (you can make yourself less vulnerable to stitch in the side by gradually increasing your workout length and intensity, and by warming up thoroughly before each workout). Doctors speculate that round ligament spasm, as it is more properly known, is caused by working out too soon after eating or an inadequate blood flow to the diaphragm and muscles to the ribs (ischemia). Exercise compels your muscles, including your respiratory muscles, to meet higher energy demands without an increased blood flow. You also breathe more frequently and deeply, further pushing these muscles.

For instant relief, stop in your tracks. Breathe in and stretch your arm directly upward on the affected side. Hold the stretch for several minutes, breathing deeply. If you still have pain after holding the stretch for two minutes, press Gall Bladder 25 and Spleen 21.

Stomach/Abdominal Discomfort

Stomach and abdominal discomfort include fullness and pressure, mild cramping, nausea, and acid indigestion (a sour feeling that permeates the stomach and upper digestive tract). You may also have diarrhea or become constipated (see the entries for Diarrhea, page 60, and Constipation, page 57). Digestive problems may be a stress response, your body's way of telling you it needs less coffee, alcohol, or spicy food.

Dietary changes are often helpful to young children who are vulnerable to stomach/abdominal discomfort. Toddlers who constantly drink fruit juice (instead of eating fresh produce) and consume few fats often have digestive problems. Pediatricians typically recommend eating a small amount of fat (such as butter or peanut butter) with each meal, and eliminating fruit or fruit-flavored drinks. Researchers successfully reduced incidences of Recurrent Abdominal Pain (RAP) in a group of six-year-olds by increasing their fiber intake. Fresh fruits, vegetables, and whole grains such as brown rice and wheat are excellent sources of fiber.

Acupressure points relax involuntary muscles in the digestive tract, quell nausea, and relieve pain. Press Spleen 3 or 4 with a strong, firm pressure as soon as you feel queasy (as in motion sickness). For prenatal morning sickness, use Triple Warmer 5. Stomach and abdominal pain also responds to Stomach 43, Stomach 45 (not to be used in pregnancy), Liver 1, and Liver 3.

Ripe, sweet grapes, thoroughly chewed, relieve an acid feeling in the mouth and stomach. Gingerroot and chamomile are common herbal remedies for indigestion. Gingerroot, which should not be used during the first six months of pregnancy, contains the enzyme zingibain, which facilitates digestion. To prepare it for children younger than ten, peel and chop 1/2 teaspoon of fresh gingerroot, then steep it in one cup of boiling water until it is cool enough to drink. This is taken a mouthful at a time throughout the day, up to a maximum of three cups per week. Adults use a whole teaspoon, and should drink five cups a week. Chamomile, an herbal tranquilizer, is also a gastrointestinal antispasmodic. In chronic cases of stomach/abdominal discomfort, chamomile tea is taken daily. To prepare it, steep one teaspoon of the dried herb in one cup of boiling water until it is cool enough to drink. Chamomile can be drunk freely by adults and children over the age of two. Infants are given half this dosage of room temperature tea in a bottle or cup.

Stress

Stress is challenge. Its source may be work demands, relationship strain, or any other situation that requires you to develop new coping mechanisms. Your psychophysical response can cause wear and tear on your body, mind, and emotions. Stress reactions are implicated in numerous health problems, including high blood pressure, headache, and depression.

Stress management begins with acknowledging it, identifying its source, and developing a stress management strategy. Acupressure, with its deeply relaxing effect, can help you reduce these negative results and stimulate you to find healthy coping mechanisms. For example, a busy attorney scheduled weekly massage appointments until a particularly difficult and drawn-out case was settled. Theater legend Helen Hayes coped with stage fright by taking short walks during intermissions. Regular acupressure self-treatment can be a welcome time-out, replacing destructive coping styles. Press Stomach 42, Heart 7 and 9, Small Intestine 10 (not to be used in pregnancy), Lung 1 and 2, and Conception Vessel 17 for stress reduction. (Also see the entries for Anxiety, page 42, and Insomnia, page 77.)

Tennis Elbow (Tendonitis)

Tennis elbow is a general term for arm stiffness and stress. It typically results from overindulgence in a favorite racquet sport, like tennis or racquetball. The pain is often described as "burning," and sometimes the arm is swollen.

Use acupressure and compresses to relieve stiffness and pain. Press Large Intestine 11, 14, and 15 for at least five minutes each. Then wrap the painful area in a very warm cloth for five minutes; following that, replace it with an ice pack. The ice pack remains for five minutes also. You can repeat the sequence as often as necessary.

When you return to your sport, take five or ten minutes of prevention time before you play. Rub, swing, and stretch the arm that is usually affected by participation in your sport. For best results, press acupressure points to further loosen your muscles and stimulate circulation.

Also see the entry for Joint Pain and Stiffness, page 78.

Testicle Torsion

Testicle torsion is a twisting pressure in the testicle that affects the spermatic cord. The blood supply to one testicle is severely reduced; this leads to cell destruction. The affected testicle reddens, swells, and throbs painfully, while the scrotum may become sensitive to touch. Nausea, sweating, and rapid heartbeat are frequent physical responses to the severe pain. Shock may also occur.

Testicle torsion seldom results from injury, and its causes are often unknown. It afflicts men of all ages but is most common in teenage boys. Testicle torsion has been noted at birth in a few instances.

This sharply painful disease always requires prompt attention at a doctor's office or emergency room. While you wait for medical treatment, apply an ice pack directly to the testicle to numb the pain. Press Acupressure points for other symptoms. (See the entries for Anxiety, page 42, Shock, page 92, and Stomach/Abdominal Discomfort, page 94.)

Toothache

Dental pain is typically caused by a carie, or cavity, literally a worn place in the tooth. Chipped or broken teeth, crowns, and fillings are usually painful, especially if a nerve is exposed as a result of the damage, and require prompt medical attention. (Do not attempt to replace crowns or fillings yourself, since this might cause further damage.) When your teeth or gums hurt, see your dentist as soon as possible. If your dentist is unavailable, call her emergency number.

Acupressure and ice packs will make you more comfortable while you wait to see your dentist. Cleanse your mouth with lukewarm water. Then press Governing Vessel 28 or Stomach 3 while you hold an ice pack over your cheek. This numbs the pain and reduces the swelling.

Tooth Grinding

See Bruxism, page 50.

Urinary Incontinence (Bed-wetting)

Children typically wet their beds while they are learning bladder control. These accidents are part of a learning process rather than a disciplinary problem. However, consult a pediatrician about a bed-wetting problem that lasts longer than three months. He should order laboratory tests to rule out kidney disease and should offer positive suggestions.

Adult bed wetters should also consult a trusted physician. If tests show that you have no urinary tract problems, the bed-wetting could be a symptom of stress overload. This can be treated with acupressure and other natural therapies.

Asian health practitioners view urinary problems as a sign of energy imbalance in the Bladder and Kidney meridians, the energy flows that serve to regulate bodily fluids. Press Kidney 3 and Bladder 64 before going to sleep. For the maximum effectiveness press points on both feet and ankles. Katie's mother pressed these points on her daughter each night after she had gone to sleep. Within a week Katie's bed-wetting had dropped by 50 percent; a month later it had disappeared.

Acupressure can be supplemented with cornsilk tea, a traditional remedy for urinary incontinence. It is made with three tablespoons of fresh cornsilk steeped in one cup of boiling water until it is cool enough to drink. Children are given a half-cup of this tea each morning; adults drink a whole cup.

Varicose Veins

Varicose ("spider") veins are swollen and painful. They usually appear in the legs, causing a dull aching that increases during exercise. A bump or blow is excruciating. Some women find that increased estrogen levels during menstruation and pregnancy intensify sensitivity.

Chinese medical caregivers press Stomach 36 (not to be used in pregnancy) and Gall Bladder 30 for quick pain relief. Continuing treatment focuses on improving circulation by toning the Fire and Water meridians. Press Heart 7 and 8, Pericardium 5, Bladder 64, Kidney 3, Small Intestine 4, and Triple Warmer 1 at least four times each week.

Constipation aggravates varicose veins in the legs; it decreases lower body circulation and increases the sensation of pressure. You can use acupressure and other natural remedies to promote healthy bowels (see the entry for Constipation, page 57).

For the maximum benefit, supplement your acupressure treatment with exercise to benefit circulation. Swimming is a safe exercise for most people with varicose veins, and many dance studios offer non-impact aerobic classes. If taught by a competent (and preferably certified) instructor, these classes give you a beneficial workout free of jumping and jogging.

Vertigo

Vertigo is an unpleasant physical sensation that includes dizziness, lack of depth and height perception, and poor balance. Nausea and vomiting sometimes accompany vertigo (see the entries for Nausea, page 84, and Vomiting, page 100). These unpleasant symptoms are often the result of another illness, such as migraine headaches and some strains of influenza (see the entries for Headache, page 70, and Influenza, page 75). Recurrent vertigo is usually the symptom of some other disease, and your doctor should be consulted.

When you have vertigo symptoms, do not drive a car or use any potentially dangerous tools such as scissors or knives. Try to stay in one place. This will keep you from falling or bumping yourself. Sit or lie quietly, and press Stomach 42, which is associated with correcting dizziness.

Vomiting

Vomiting occurs when your stomach rejects a substance that it doesn't need at the moment. This problem can result from a variety of causes such as overeating, overdrinking, nervousness, or emotional upset (see the entry for Anxiety, page 42). Nausea and vomiting are also strongly associated with stomach-affecting viral diseases such as influenza (see the entry for Influenza, page 75).

Press Spleen 3 and Stomach 42 for prompt relief of vomiting, since the Earth meridians regulate the digestive organs.

When you vomit, you are subject to dehydration (water loss). Dehydration also depletes your body of essential salts. (It is a particularly hazardous condition for infants.) Symptoms include dry mouth and a sudden decrease in urination. Replenish your water supply with clear liquids like ice water and tea. Cooled mint teas are sometimes soothing to a sore, tired digestive system. Steep one teaspoon of spearmint or peppermint tea in one cup of boiling water and cool it in a refrigerator or freezer. (The cooled tea can also be put in a baby's bottle.) Mint teas may be drunk freely.

Also see the entries for Dehydration, page 111, Nausea, page 84, and Stomach/Abdominal Discomfort, page 94.

Whiplash

Whiplash is the common name for an upper-body injury normally suffered in a car accident. When your car is struck from behind, the impact abruptly jerks your head and neck. (If you suffered a head injury, you must see a doctor promptly.) This creates stiffness and stress in the muscles of your upper back, neck, and shoulders, which can last for days, weeks, or months after the accident. It is naturally aggravated by the emotional stress of suffering accident and injury.

You may be able to prevent some whiplash aftereffects by

promptly treating the affected area with acupressure. Once it has been conclusively determined that you have not suffered an upper-body fracture or wound that would be aggravated by pressure, you can press points to relax tight muscles, stimulate circulation, and encourage emotional release. Press Bladder 38, Large Intestine 14 and 15, Small Intestine 11, Gall Bladder 21, and Governing Vessel 13 and 15 to release neck and upper-back tension. A scalp massage is also helpful. For emotional release and eventual calming, press Lung 1 and 2, Conception Vessel 17, and Heart 7, 8, and 9.

Yeast Infection

See Monilia, page 83.

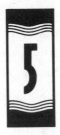

Acupressure for Infants
and Children

Acupressure has particular benefits for infants and young people. My practice includes children with ear infection, hyperactivity, and bed-wetting. I find acupressure helpful for relief of the fever, restlessness, and itching associated with "kid's diseases" such as measles, mumps, and chicken pox.

Acupressure is a good skill to learn for parents and friends of children. Timely, sensitive touch can soothe a panicked or sleepless child, and communicate love and protection. Maggie pressed acupressure points to relieve her six-year-old daughter's insomnia during a family crisis. Touch can also be a way to reach older children who are struggling to develop autonomy. Dylan, age twelve, was upset and angry over a school problem he was eager to solve independently. His mother offered him a foot massage, telling him he would think more clearly if he was relaxed. Somewhat to her surprise, Dylan accepted. After she rubbed and pressed for a few moments, he began to talk about the difficulty, and found himself willing to accept her feedback.

Dylan's mother displayed commendable sensitivity, an important tool for working with young people. There are special considerations for giving touch therapies to children, particularly if they do not know you well. A child needs to understand from the beginning that you don't give shots. (If you practice in a medical office, avoid wearing a laboratory coat; these signal "needle" to preschoolers.) Explain what acupressure does and what it feels like. You can say something like, "Pressing this point balances you, so you feel relaxed and calm, and this will help your headache."

Sometimes a child will say, "Don't touch me." Something about you may have frightened her, or she could be practicing new self-assertion skills. Treat this respectfully; she's learning to protect herself from unsafe touch. You can respond by saying, "It's really great that you can tell me what you want like that. But I can't help you with the itching if I don't touch you—I'll be very careful." Persuade, don't force.

Keep sessions short, since they will bore most young children. Music or a story (read aloud by another adult or an older child) keep a child still while you press points. You can also press points while they're sleeping. However, children sometimes need to move around when tension releases. I treated Star, age five, for frequent ear infections. After I pressed Small Intestine 4 for three minutes, she got up from the futon and began stretching. I was astonished to see her move naturally into classic hatha yoga positions.

Bed-wetting

See Urinary Incontinence, page 98.

Blood on Underwear or Diaper

See Anal Fissure, page 42.

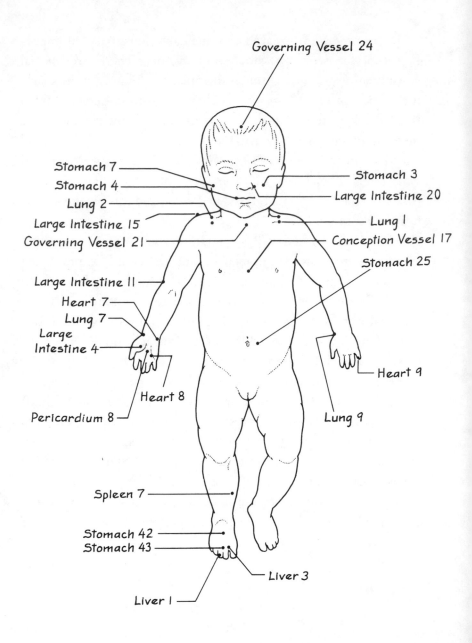

Governing Vessel 24

Stomach 7
Stomach 4
Lung 2
Large Intestine 15
Governing Vessel 21

Stomach 3
Large Intestine 20
Lung 1
Conception Vessel 17
Stomach 25

Large Intestine 11
Heart 7
Lung 7
Large Intestine 4

Heart 9

Pericardium 8

Heart 8

Lung 9

Spleen 7

Stomach 42
Stomach 43

Liver 3

Liver 1

**Acupressure Points
on an Infant**

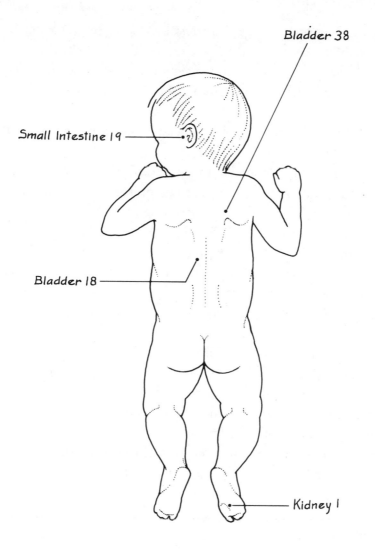

Bladder 38

Small Intestine 19

Bladder 18

Kidney 1

Breast-feeding Problems

To breast-feed successfully, you must be able to release a steady flow of milk. Acupressure helps you do this by relaxing you, encouraging the essential milk ejection reflex. Your pituitary gland secretes oxytocin, a hormone that stimulates your breasts to let down milk. The oxytocin release, with its subsequent release of milk for your baby, is blocked when you are tense. If your breasts become engorged, relax in a warm bath and press Lung 1, Kidney 22, Stomach 13 and 16, Gall Bladder 20, and Liver 3. You can also apply warm compresses to your breasts.

Rub a chemical-free oil (see Resources, page 131) into your nipples at least twice a day while you're nursing. This prevents drying and cracking. If your nipple cracks, be certain to keep it very clean. You will probably want to hand-express your milk and give it to your baby in a bottle while the sore nipple heals. Use a cotton swab to dab aloe vera gel on the broken skin every half-hour or so.

Help prevent nursing difficulties by taking good care of yourself. You must acknowledge that breastfeeding is a major demand on your body, and poor nutrition and fatigue will sabotage your efforts. Take a vitamin supplement specifically designed for nursing mothers, along with two grams of calcium each day. Learn to prioritize your time, and enlist the help of your partner, relatives, and friends to be sure that you get enough rest.

Chicken Pox

Chicken pox, which originates with the herpes zoster virus, is identified by blisterlike skin eruptions. After about twenty-four hours, these collapse and form scabs. Accompanying fever and sweating make the patient itchily uncomfortable. (Do not give children aspirin for the fever. Aspirin use during viral infections is strongly associated with Reye's Syndrome, a potentially fatal disease that strikes young people under eighteen. See page 109.)

Chicken pox has no lasting results for most people. However, if the scabs are scratched, they could become infected. Explain this to your child, and keep her fingernails short to discourage scratching. You can also use acupressure and other natural remedies to relieve the heat and itching. Glen gave his daughter twice daily acupressure sessions. He began with a cool compress on her forehead, to make her less feverish, and pressed Spleen 7 to relieve the itching. (When symptoms were acute, it sometimes took as long as seven minutes before Glen felt the point pulsate evenly.) He continued by pressing points on the Metal meridians, since these govern skin health.

For your own chicken pox treatments, follow Spleen 7 with three or more of the following points: Large Intestine 1, 4 (forbidden in pregnancy), 11, and 20 and Lung 1, 2, 7, and 9. Also see the entries for Fever, page 66, and Stress, page 95.

Children usually recover completely in a week or ten days, while adults tend to have symptoms lasting for several weeks. Children and adults need to stay indoors, away from friends and family who have never had this contagious disease. (Once you've had chicken pox you're immune to the herpes zoster virus, which also causes shingles in adults.)

Colic

Colic is a series of painful intestinal spasms. It is most common in babies from birth to three months of age.

Europeans use a mild herbal tea to soothe colic pain. Steep one-half teaspoon of dried fennel leaves in one cup of boiling water until it is cool, then give it to your baby in a bottle.

When she finishes, rock her or walk with her in your arms. Sing and talk reassuringly, telling her that you know she hurts and that you want her to feel better soon.

Convulsions

Convulsions are most common in children under two years of age, although they can occur in children as old as six. They typically occur in response to fever (see the entry for Fever, page 66). Young children are highly sensitive to rapid elevations of heat, since the temperature-regulating brainstem does not mature until age four. If a child's temperature rises too rapidly, convulsions may result. Since convulsions are a medical emergency, call a doctor or emergency room as soon as your child regains consciousness.

During a convulsion, your child is unconscious and cannot respond to you. Since his entire muscular system is engaged, his whole body is affected. His limbs are stiff and his back arches. His eyes move rapidly. Throat spasms prevent him from swallowing saliva, so that he appears to be frothing at the mouth. If his seizure lasts for more than one to two minutes, his skin may become blue from the loss of oxygen.

During a convulsion, your first concern is to keep your child from injuring himself. Make sure he can't knock against hard furniture. Remove him from a bed or sofa to the floor, or to a crib, so he can't fall. Place a clean cloth between his teeth to keep him from biting his tongue. Try to keep a comforting hand on your child so that it's the first thing he's aware of when he becomes conscious; continually attempt to establish eye contact. This will

---

A MEDICAL EMERGENCY

Your child needs immediate medical attention at a doctor's office or emergency room if his breathing is difficult or rapid (eighty or more inhalations per minute) or his lips or nails turn blue.

---

help you to determine when he can respond to you again and the convulsion is over.

Your child will recover more rapidly if you stay as calm as possible. Reassure him for a moment, and then tell him that you need a doctor to help take care of him.

After you call the doctor, try to find another adult to drive you to his office or an emergency room. Hold your child during the drive. Talk reassuringly, sing, and massage his hands and feet to relax and reassure him. Press Heart 7, 8, and 9, Pericardium 8, and Stomach 45 to further calm your child. Stay with him during the medical examination, and follow the doctor's instructions carefully and completely.

Cradle Cap

Cradle cap is a thick yellow or yellowish-white crust that appears on the top of an infant's head. This is a symptom of seborrheic

---

REYE'S SYNDROME

Reye's Syndrome is a form of encephalitis, which afflicts infants and young people under age eighteen. It is potentially fatal, and survivors are likely to suffer coma or permanent brain damage. Research links RS with aspirin use when viral infections, particularly chicken pox and flu, are present.

If your child shows any of these early RS symptoms, he requires immediate medical attention at a doctor's office or emergency room:

mental confusion

lethargy

double vision

weakness or paralysis in arms and legs

hearing loss

speech impairment

---

dermatitis, not a lack of cleanliness. Fortunately, cradle cap isn't painful or itchy. Some children have it periodically until age three, particularly in humid climates. Cradle cap is not connected with the hair loss that is natural for some infants at three and four months of age.

Cradle cap is aggravated by baby-care products that contain alcohol (read labels!). Replace these with a mild shampoo or use soap bulb (see Resources, page 131). Brush your baby's hair several times daily with a soft-bristled brush.

For stubborn cases of cradle cap, gently rub a warm, wet washcloth over his scalp before brushing. This softens the crust and makes removal easier.

Croup

Croup is a bacterial or viral infection common to infants and preschoolers. Your child's throat, vocal cords, and bronchial tubes are swollen and inflamed. Her breath is probably labored, and she has a barking cough. This is very uncomfortable and frightening for her. Your reassuring attention and touch can do a great deal to relax her and make breathing easier (for you both!).

Turn a hot shower on full force and close the bathroom door and windows while the room fills with steam. Improvise a futon with blankets, thick towels, or sleeping bags for your child. Then talk and sing to her while you press Bladder 18, Lung 1, Lung 2, Stomach 7, Conception Vessel 17 and 21, and Governing Vessel 24. This treatment will be most effective if you are calm and reassuring.

Continue pressing at least four points each day for one week after a croup attack. Pediatricians recommend placing a cool-mist humidifier in her bedroom during this period. Inhaling the mist while she sleeps will help keep her respiratory tract clear so she can breathe easily.

Also see the entries for Asthma, page 44, and Colds and Bronchitis, page 54.

Dehydration

Dehydration means a water loss, and the subsequent depletion of body salts. It can affect people of all ages, but this is a particularly dangerous condition for an infant. Dehydration symptoms including dry mouth, wrinkled skin, and a sudden decrease in urination may follow a bout of vomiting or diarrhea (see the entries for Diarrhea, page 60, and Stomach/Abdominal Discomfort, page 94) or overexposure to hot weather. These symptoms must be monitored by your pediatrician; follow her instructions carefully.

Press Kidney 1 to strengthen your baby's Water meridians, and give your baby cool liquids every half hour; Gatorade and licorice root tea are often used to restore fluid balance. (Gatorade, a commercial soft drink, is popular with athletes who constantly lose water through sweating.) Dried licorice root can be purchased at a health food store or ordered from a catalog (see Resources, page 131). For your baby, steep one teaspoon of the herb in three cups of boiling water until the water reaches room temperature. Then refrigerate it until it is cool. Let your baby drink as much as he likes.

THE TOUCH-SENSITIVE INFANT

A few babies display a limited tolerance for touching and holding. Cuddling doesn't comfort them when they are fussy or tired. This is often frustrating or worrisome to the new parent. Relax. Your baby isn't rejecting you; she's communicating her unique needs. Baby care experts recognize that some infants are easily overstimulated by touch.

However, the touch-sensitive baby still needs to bond with you just like any other infant. Cuddle her on a folded blanket or pillow, or let her lie on her back in her crib while you talk, sing, and maintain eye contact. She will deeply appreciate your sensitivity.

In hot weather, be especially careful to give your baby plenty of liquids and keep him cool. When he's not out in the sun, let him wear as few clothes as possible. You can sponge him frequently with cool water, and some infants and toddlers love to be squirted with a plant mister when it's hot.

Diaper Rash (Prickly Heat)

Diaper rash is a common problem with infants. Its causes include too infrequent diaper changes, chemical sensitivities, and water-proof pants. These keep the skin wet with urine, causing irritation. Begin your baby's treatment by taking a hard look at your laundry detergents and baby-care products. You can substitute additive-free lotions, soaps, and powders for the baby care products found in most supermarkets or drugstores. Jojoba, a cactus product, makes a fine baby oil. You can substitute fine white clay for manufactured baby powder. Soap bulb, if it grows in your area, is a gentle natural cleanser for skin and hair. Most manufacturers of natural-health products will send you a free catalog (see Resources, page 131).

Rebecca found that her son's diaper rash diminished when she pressed Spleen 7 and Liver 3 during his afternoon nap. She also tried cutting the amount of detergent she used in his laundry by one half, and added a cup of vinegar to her washer at the start of the rinse cycle. This neutralized the detergent residue, and the rash, as well as his subsequent irritability, disappeared within three days.

For short-term relief, press acupressure points while you hold and talk to your baby. Spleen 7 relieves itching, and the Metal meridians strengthen the skin. Touch Lung 1 and 7 and Large Intestine 1, 4, and 11. Use particularly gradual and gentle pressure with your baby. Always stop pressing if it seems to distress him.

You can also rub aloe vera gel into the rash to give him some relief from its heat.

Earaches

See Ear Discomfort, page 61.

Headache

See page 70.

Hyperventilation

Hyperventilation is breathing that is too rapid. It decreases the carbon dioxide levels in the blood, altering blood chemistry and affecting the central nervous system. This in turn causes symptoms such as muscle spasms, weakness, and sometimes fainting. (See the entry for Fainting, page 65.) Hyperventilation can accompany severe illness or injury, but is more commonly caused by an "I can't cope" feeling. Frequent hyperventilation should be discussed with a pediatrician.

When your child hyperventilates, promptly press Lung 1. You can also distract him by asking him to help you with point location, and then have him press Lung 1 on both sides while you press Conception Vessel 17, Bladder 38, Heart 8, and Pericardium 8.

Just as a sniffle can signal an oncoming cold, hyperventilation is often a symptom of an underlying trauma or worry. Nancy was savagely attacked by a wandering dog at age four and suffered facial wounds that required surgery. After her hospital discharge, she began hyperventilating at the sight of a dog, leashed or unleashed, and suffered from nightmares. A family counselor encouraged Nancy's parents to act out the trauma with dolls and stuffed animals and to draw pictures. Although this process took many months, eventually Nancy's trauma eased and her symptoms disappeared.

Impetigo (Pyoderma)

Impetigo is a skin infection caused by staphylococci or streptococci bacteria. This vivid red rash usually is seen in toddlers and preschoolers, and fair-skinned children seem most susceptible. A few impetigo patients also develop a low-grade fever (see the entry for Fever, page 66). An infection consists of numerous pus-filled blisters that break easily and form yellow crusts. The rash is extremely itchy, and scratching will spread it. Explain this to your child, and keep her fingernails short to avoid scratching.

With prompt diagnosis and treatment, impetigo should resolve in five to ten days. While your child rests or naps, press Spleen 7 to relieve the itching. Then press Liver 1 and 3 and Large Intestine 4 and 11, since each of these points affects skin health. Remember to wash your hands if you accidentally touch the rash while giving acupressure treatment. Impetigo is extremely contagious! Make sure everyone in your household uses their own washcloth and towel until the rash disappears, and stays that way, for at least two days. A child with impetigo must not sleep with other family members until she is completely well.

Your doctor can prescribe oral antibiotics or antibiotic cream. Follow his instructions carefully. In addition, wash the rash at least three times daily with antibacterial soap. Use paper towels to scrub away the crust, exposing the blisters (see the entry for Blisters, page 48), before you cover it with a bandage. Then discard the paper towels and wash your hands thoroughly.

Measles

Measles is a viral illness that affects the skin, mucous membranes, and respiratory tract. It is extremely contagious.

Pregnant women who do not recall receiving a physician's diagnosis of rubella should not take care of someone with measles symptoms. This measles strain was shown to cause birth defects.

Measles' most visible symptom is a red rash, and sometimes white spots inside the mouth and throat. Some patients get a runny nose and cough. Measles sufferers are tired, have little appetite, and generally run a temperature of about 102 degrees. Their eyes are reddish and are sensitive to light. Do not give aspirin to children for symptom relief, since its use with measles is associated with Reye's Syndrome (see page 109).

You can use acupressure to relieve measles symptoms that include itching, fatigue, and eye irritation. See the entries for Colds and Bronchitis, page 54, Contact Dermatitis, page 58, Eyestrain, page 64, and Fatigue, page 65.

Mumps

Mumps is a mild viral disease most common in children between the ages of two and twelve. The salivary glands, located between the ear and jaw, are sore. Mumps patients need to be isolated and watched for abdominal pain, severe headache, and swollen, painful testicles. These symptoms indicate the need for a pediatrician's care.

Acupressure can relieve mumps symptoms. Gently press Stomach 6 on both sides of the jaw to relieve tension and promote healthy circulation. Refer to the entries for Bruxism, page 50, Fever, page 66, and Pharyngitis, page 87.

Nosebleed

Most children suffer a few nosebleeds in the course of ordinary play. These can be stopped within minutes. Pinch the nostrils together lightly and direct the child to breathe through his mouth without swallowing blood, since this will make him nauseated. If you have some ice on hand, wrap one cube in a plastic bag and hold this against either side of the nose.

The bleeding will stop when a clot forms inside the nose. (If this takes longer than ten minutes, call your pediatrician.) Tell the child not to blow his nose for about twelve hours, since this will disturb the clot and start the bleeding again.

If your child suffers from nosebleeds more than three times a year, discuss the problem with a physician. A laboratory test can show whether the blood loss has caused anemia. A doctor can order other tests to determine whether the nosebleeds indicate a more serious underlying problem.

Penis Irritation

See Balanitis, page 45.

Poison Exposure or Ingestion

See page 88.

Poison Oak, Ivy, or Sumac

See page 89.

Stomachache

See Stomach/Abdominal Discomfort, page 94.

Teething

Teething babies are afflicted with pain, excess saliva production, and irritability. Most begin teething at six months of age, when the lower front teeth normally appear. Teething may continue up to age three and a half. A similar pain may also occur when the first adult teeth come in (about age six). There may also be pain when the bicuspids, or side teeth, show up in late childhood, and when permanent molars appear at puberty.

Occasionally, a spot of blood appears at the site of a burgeoning tooth. Consult your dentist if the spot becomes large or remains longer than three days.

Massaging the gums provides relief and stimulates healthful circulation. Rub with a clean index finger and press Stomach 3 and 4, traditionally used to relieve dental pain. Another classic remedy is to numb the gums with whiskey or gin. Use the smallest amount possible for relief; children should not consume liquor.

Ice also numbs sore gums. You can freeze a washcloth (be sure it's too large for her to swallow) and let your toddler chew it.

Tonsillitis

Tonsillitis is an infection of the tonsils, small masses of lymphoid tissue at the back of your throat. It is caused by a virus or by harmful bacteria. Children and adults with tonsillitis suffer ear and throat pain and have swollen lymph glands for about three days. A few patients have a cough, and nearly all suffer from headaches. (Children under eighteen should not take aspirin for relief, since its use in viral infections is associated with Reye's Syndrome. See page 109.) A pediatrician can determine if the infection is caused by streptococcal bacteria, and will prescribe antibiotics if necessary.

Tonsillitis sufferers should rest in bed, drink mint teas to soothe the throat, and use acupressure. Refer to Ear Discomfort, page 61, Headache, page 70, Stress, page 95, and Pharyngitis, page 87.

Umbilical Cord Infection

A baby's umbilical stump normally withers and drops off the navel within ten days of birth. Let this happen naturally without twisting or pulling, which makes a painful bacterial infection likely. Wash the stump and navel thoroughly at each diaper change, since it probably gets soaked in urine.

An infected umbilical stump oozes yellow fluid that crusts. The surrounding area may also be swollen and red. If these symptoms appear, promptly contact your obstetrical caregiver. Follow her instructions carefully, and make certain that the cord is clean and covered at all times. After you wash it, use a sterile cotton swab to dab soothing aloe vera gel on the affected area. Then hug your baby and reassure him that he will soon feel fine.

Vaginal Discharge and Itching

Prepubertal girls are subject to nonspecific vaginitis, an irritation that manifests without apparent cause. Before puberty the vaginal walls are thin and easily affected by bacteria. If your daughter complains of itching and painful urination, she may have an infection. She may also have some vaginal discharge. These symptoms can result from an allergy to colored toilet paper or detergent soaps. Other causes include insufficient cleanliness or the insertion of an object (such as a bead) into this interesting orifice. She may also have contracted yeast from a washcloth or towel (see the entry for Monilia, page 83).

Press Spleen 7 to give her some immediate relief from the itching, and discuss the importance of keeping her vaginal area very clean. Replace your colored toilet paper with an uncolored product (see Resources, page 131).

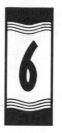

Acupressure for People Sixty or Better

My "sixty-or-better" clients have much to gain from acupressure. While most of their health concerns are similar to younger people's, they do have particular considerations, including joint stiffness and circulation. Women especially ask about strengthening the bladder (see the entry for Bladder Symptoms, page 46). I often press Liver 3, Lung 7, and Triple Warmer 3 on older clients to strengthen their resistance to disease, since their recovery time tends to be lengthier than younger people's. I have treated several wheelchair users for low back pain. Whatever your age or state of health, you can benefit from acupressure's deeply relaxing effects. If you are frequently ill or disabled, ask a relative or caretaker to press points for you. They should read this chapter before doing so.

You can learn to press points on yourself for the prevention and relief of everyday discomfort. For the maximum benefit, spend at least fifteen to thirty minutes each day pressing points. Make this part of your daily routine; for example, press points before you get out of bed in the morning. If you regularly take time to relax during the day, start with acupressure self-treatment. This will leave you even more refreshed than usual. You are more likely to press points consistently if acupressure self-care is a regular part of your life.

AN ACUPRESSURE SELF-TREATMENT SESSION

Start with a few deep, relaxed breaths, or go through A Calming Meditation on page 43. Then think about what you would like to get from this self-care session.

It's always helpful to begin with one or two points that facilitate overall relaxation. Press Lung 1 and 2, Conception Vessel 17, or Heart 7 and 8. (Also see the entries for Anxiety, page 42, and Stress, page 95.) Daily preventive maintenance for your joints is also a good idea (see the entry for Joint Pain and Stiffness, page 78). If you have a particular health concern, turn to the appropriate section and press the points indicated.

Complete your session by strengthening the meridians that govern your immune system. Use one or more of these points: Triple Warmer 3 and 5; Large Intestine 11; Lung 1, 2, and 7; and Liver 3. Then rest quietly.

You will always get the best results from acupressure when you combine it with proper nutrition, age-appropriate exercise, and an interest in life. If you feel victimized by your age or by health problems, your best responses are positive thinking and direct, constructive action. Join special-interest groups such as the American Association of Retired Persons (AARP) and the Grey Panthers; these groups work on your behalf.

You can contribute substantially to your good health by using your time and mind positively. Research has established that memory loss is usually caused by too little physical and mental exercise. Much "senility" results from isolation or the side effects of painkillers and sedatives. When your doctor agrees, substitute acupressure for potentially numbing drugs, or press points to minimize side effects like fatigue and confusion (see the entries for Fatigue, page 65, and Stress, page 95).

Be creative and resourceful in deciding where and how you want to contribute. There are many opportunities for service. Some employers rehire former workers on a part-time or consulting basis. Grace, a former laboratory supervisor, took her younger replacement's suggestion that she return to work on special projects three days per week. Volunteer work is another possibility. Upon retirement from the White House, Jimmy and Rosalyn Carter became volunteer construction workers with Habitat for Humanity. They built homes in inner cities, working alongside the low-income families who would eventually own them.

Evaluate your time, energy, and talents to determine where you can contribute. You have never had this much knowledge, skill, and mature perspective. The world needs these qualities— it needs you, at your healthy, active best.

Menopausal Symptoms

Menopause, literally the cessation of menstruation, typically occurs between the ages of forty-five and fifty-five. It is incomplete until you have missed twelve consecutive menstrual periods. During menopause your ovaries slow down their usual production of estrogen, and some women have uncomfortable symptoms. These typically include bladder problems such as incontinence (see Bladder Symptoms, page 46), and hot flashes.

Hot flashes are painless rushes of heat that suffuse your upper body for a few seconds up to two minutes. They may appear several times an hour or several times a day. They are most common in the evening, when body temperature peaks. Sometimes hot flashes and sweating wake you up at night. Alcohol and coffee make you warm and seem to increase the frequency of the episodes in some women.

Asian medical practitioners treat hot flashes by pressing cooling points to balance body temperatures. If they are a daily occurrence, press Stomach 42 twice each day. Supplement these points with Triple Warmer 3, Kidney 3, and Bladder 66 if hot flashes are a frequent problem.

Acupressure for Wheelchair Users

If you use a wheelchair, you must pay special attention to preventing lower back pain and stimulating lower body circulation. Press Governing Vessel 2 and 4 and Bladder 42 faithfully each day. Supplement these points with Gall Bladder 30, Governing Vessel 12, Bladder 47, Bladder 38, and Triple Warmer 15 on days when you feel particularly stiff. If you find it difficult to reach these points while sitting upright, lie on a firm mattress and place tennis balls beneath the points. Use new tennis balls to get sufficient pressure to promote relaxed muscles and efficient circulation.

Also see Back Pain and Tension, page 44, Cold Hands and Feet, page 53, and Joint Pain and Stiffness, page 78.

For the maximum comfort, move, stretch, and bend as much as you can throughout the day. Stretch your neck. Rotate your arms and bend and sway forward and sideways. This strengthens your muscles and stimulates healthy circulation.

Finally, make certain that your wheelchair fits you properly. Experiment with different sizes and styles to find what's most comfortable for you. Give your lower back some extra support by propping a small pillow or rolled-up blanket at the base of your spine. Check with medical supply houses that carry a wide variety of foam and plastic wheelchair aids.

Acupressure for Disabled or Frail Elderly People

Disabled or frail elderly people need light pressure, since they bruise easily. Press into points very gradually, and watch their faces carefully for their responses to your pressure and depth.

Many people with limited mobility are isolated, so they are tragically unused to caring touch and attention. They often talk compulsively during acupressure sessions; encourage this important tension release. (Other outlets, like vigorous exercise, are not available to them.) Some lose track of their original subject and ramble confusedly for a few minutes. However, respectful attention is the appropriate response, even when you don't understand them completely. Early in my practice, I learned that elderly clients always responded to careful listening. Rambling invariably subsided into a coherent description of their needs, concerns, and unfinished business. Nahum, a retired textile importer, shared a particularly moving example of unfinished business during a session.

Nahum originally came to acupressure for arthritis relief. I taught him to press Bladder 48 and Gall Bladder 30 for hip tension, and we used reflexology to increase dexterity in his hands. We saw each other weekly for several months until he was hospitalized for a hip replacement operation. We scheduled a session for several days after his hospital discharge.

When I met Nahum at his apartment, he seemed subdued and vacant. As soon as he lay down for acupressure, however, he began to talk compulsively. As I pressed Small Intestine 11, his topics ranged from a long-ago trip to Shanghai to his time in the hospital to his plans for an upcoming holiday—often all in the same sentence. This continued for nearly ten minutes. Then Nahum took a deep breath, and his face relaxed. He began to speak in clear, chilling detail about his family's incarceration in a Nazi concentration camp during World War II. I quietly pressed Lung 1 and Bladder 38 for emotional release, and the horrors spilled out. "We were prisoners, and there was no help. No doctor for any of us. Someone would have a toothache, and it would get worse, and then maybe they would die." When we finished, he said, "I am sorry I hit my children so hard, but I had to make them eat. I wanted them to stay alive. I must tell them— I must tell them this, very soon."

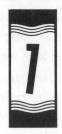

Supplements to Acupressure

Acupressure can be supplemented with natural products, exercise, and mental imagery for maximum symptom relief. You also need to find alternatives to finger pressure when it would cause further pain or damage. Herbs and aloe vera gel are helpful with some kinds of injury and illness. Yoga, stretching, and other gentle exercises ease stiff muscles and stimulate circulation. Visualization and affirmations are mental techniques that promote positive mental images to complement treatment.

Natural therapies are safe and helpful when used properly. Follow the instructions for these remedies just as carefully as you follow the directions printed on a prescription bottle; misapplication can render treatment ineffective or even harmful.

HERBALISM

Herbs were the first medicines and they are still widely used. Plant medicines are components of some prescription drugs manufactured in North America. They are also taken in pure form. German physicians routinely treat aggressive personality disorders and child hyperactivity with valerian root. European researchers verified its strong sedative effects and found that subjects exhibited none of the clumsiness and confusion associated with prescription tranquilizers. (Several subjects demonstrated enhanced problem-solving and motor skills after ingesting valerian root.)

Holistically oriented health professionals and laypeople increasingly consider herbs to be an alternative to some kinds of prescription medication. There are herbal digestive remedies, skin-care aids, and tonics for anemia, to name only a few. You can keep herbs in your home health kit for many everyday needs.

Purchase herbs from a reputable dealer or grow them yourself

YOUR HOME HEALTH KIT

Herbs

Comfrey, chamomile, goldenseal (not used in pregnancy), boneset, echinacea.

Other Natural Products

Powdered clay, aloe vera gel, ice
Bandages
Unbleached muslin, sterile Band-Aids, gauze pads, and elastic bandages in assorted sizes

Tools

Mortar and pestle, small scissors, sterile cotton pads

Telephone Numbers

Your doctor, dentist, ambulance, police, poison control, fire department

to ensure proper identification. It is often difficult to match plants to drawings, photographs, or your memory, since they vary in appearance throughout the year. Correct identification is essential since some herbs are poisonous. Fennel, a mild digestive tonic, looks only slightly different from its neighbor hemlock, the poison that killed Socrates.

HERBAL REMEDIES

Teas

To make an herbal tea, measure the required amount of dried herb into a teaball or strainer (follow specific directions for each herb) and steep this in a cup of boiling water until it is cool enough to drink. Use pure or bottled water, as chemically treated water may deplete the herbs' active ingredients.

Poultices

Cut a clean piece of unbleached muslin twice the size of the injury to be treated. Place one to three tablespoons of the herb in the cloth, fold the cloth over, and pour hot water from a teakettle over the covered herb. When the poultice is cool enough to touch, apply it directly to the wound. Loosely wrap an elastic bandage around the poultice to keep it in place during transport.

Pastes

Place two or three tablespoons of the powdered herb in a bowl. Add boiling water, one tablespoon at a time, stirring, until the mixture is firm. Apply directly to a rash or insect sting with clean hands. Do not rub it over unaffected skin; this spreads the infection. Let the paste dry completely (this will take about half an hour), then rinse it off.

Be sure to purchase herbs that are clean and free of harmful additives. Some dried herbs contain ash and dirt; chemical analysis has shown others to be laced with pesticides. Still others are bottled in alcohol tincture, which destroys the active ingredients.

Herbs are most effective when fresh (or freshly dried). Buy them in small quantities and replace the unused herbs in your home health kit every six months. Store them in tightly covered jars, kept in a closed cupboard, to delay drying of volatile oils. Used herbs should be discarded in a compost heap or garbage pail.

NATURAL PRODUCTS

Aloe vera gel has a place in your home health kit, since it is said to stimulate tissue restoration. It is more commonly used to soothe heat injuries such as sunburn, as a moisturizer for dry skin, and as a salve for wounds. It is applied directly to affected skin with a sterile cotton pad.

Aloe vera is most effective in its pure gel form, so check the label to make sure that only a little water has been added.

Use the gel rather than fresh leaves from an aloe plant, since they contain chlorophyll, which sometimes stings.

Clay is a skin tonic that tightens, cleanses, and promotes surface circulation. Clay facial masks are used to treat acne and skin wrinkling. Clay masks are also applied to wounds, bunions, and corns.

Clay is purchased at health food stores in powdered form. It comes in several different colors, each used for a different skin type. Light green clay is generally used by people with dry or aging skin, while oily skin is treated with red and black clays.

Prepare the clay just before its use; it dries quickly. Use a mortar and pestle to grind the clay into a fine powder, then place the powdered clay in a bowl. Dampen it with water and stir to make a paste that is applied directly to your skin, where it takes about half an hour to dry. Then remove the dried clay with wet paper towels or wash it off with a garden hose, letting it fall onto a lawn or flower bed where it won't clog household drains. Clay is not to be reused.

Ice is used to prevent swelling and the hemorrhaging that leads to bruising. It also numbs pain from muscle strain and sprains and wounds such as insect bites and stings.

Ice can be kept handy in a freezer or a picnic cooler. Use plastic bags to make a durable ice pack. Put one bag inside the other (a double layer minimizes tearing) and fill with ice. This is applied directly to the affected area.

STRETCHING

Movement can be very helpful for muscular problems, especially those resulting from inactivity. Some muscular discomfort is prevented with a regular exercise program that emphasizes adequate stretching during warm-up and cool-down periods.

The stretches shown on page 129 will help you to develop a routine that meets your needs.

Before you begin these stretches (or any other exercise!), warm up gently and slowly. Stretch only as far as you can manage comfortably. Your range will extend with regular stretching. Be especially careful about this if you have an injury.

USE YOUR MIND

You can encourage the healing process by courting strong, positive thoughts and images that leave you feeling optimistic and relaxed. Affirmations and visualizations are mental healing tools used for this purpose.

Foster a healing frame of mind with affirmations, strong positive statements that confirm and strengthen your faith in your healing process. Examples: "My shoulder feels flexible and free." "I process depression quickly and effectively." "It is easy for me to relax." This expands your capacity for hope, a great healing tool.

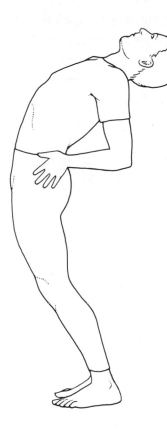

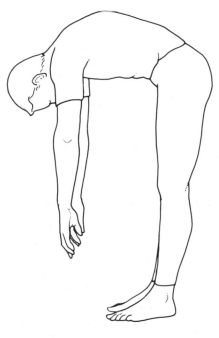

Stretching Exercises

You can also practice visualization, the formation of mental images. Create a detailed mental image of yourself looking, acting, and feeling well and strong; for the maximum benefit, do this several times a day. John came to acupressure for the treatment of tennis elbow, a condition that involves arm stiffness and pain. He learned to visualize his shoulder and elbow joints moving smoothly and painlessly. John imagined himself playing tennis and lifting weights without stress or strain. He also pressed Large Intestine 11 twice daily, and temporarily limited his tennis court time. Within three weeks of beginning treatment and supplementary self-care, John was back on the tennis courts every day.

Resources

PRODUCTS

Bronson Pharmaceuticals
4526 Rinetti Lane
P.O. Box 628
La Cañada, California 91012–0628
818–790–2646

Write or call for their free catalog of nutritional supplements and additive-free cosmetic products such as jojoba oil.

New American Food Company
2833 Duke Homestead
Durham, North Carolina 27705
1–800–835–2246

Send $1.00 for their catalog of natural foods, herbs and spices, and skin- and baby-care supplies.

Ecco-Bella
Six Provost Square, Suite 602
Caldwell, New Jersey 07006
1–800–888–5320
In New Jersey, call 201–226–5799.

Write or call for their free catalog of irritant-free body care products, household cleansers, and recycled paper products.

PERIODICALS

American Health: Fitness of Body and Mind
RD Publications, Inc.
28 West 23rd Street
New York, New York 10010

This monthly magazine addresses contemporary health issues with a refreshingly open-minded yet responsible approach.

Massage Magazine
P.O. Box 1389
Kailua-Kona, Hawaii 96745

Massage Magazine is issued bimonthly. It includes discussions of bodywork schools and styles, examples of touch therapy practice, and holistic health legalities.

The Herb Companion
306 North Washington Avenue
Loveland, Colorado 80537

This attractive bimonthly magazine features herbal cultivation methods, remedies, recipes, and crafts.

BOOKS

Bauer, Cathryn. *Acupressure for Women*. Freedom, CA: The Crossing Press, 1987. A guide for acupressure self-treatment of women's health problems.

Cousins, Norman. *Anatomy of an Illness.* New York, NY: W. W. Norton and Co. Inc., 1979. The story of a cancer patient who took charge of his own healing process.

Gardner, Joy. *The New Healing Yourself.* Freedom, CA: The Crossing Press, 1989. A compendium of herbal remedies.

Griffith, H. Winter, M.D. *Complete Guide to Pediatric Symptoms, Illness, and Medications.* Los Angeles, California: The Body Press, 1989. A reference text on young people's health problems from birth through adolescence.

Elson M. Haas, M.D. *Staying Healthy with the Seasons.* Berkeley, CA: Celestial Arts, 1981. A guide for healthy living throughout the year, containing recipes and recommendations for living according to the Five Elements Theory.

Kunz, Kevin, and Kunz, Barbara. *The Complete Guide to Foot Reflexology.* Englewood Cliffs, NJ: Prentice Hall, Inc., 1980. A handbook for practicing foot massage.

Nickel, David J. *Acupressure for Athletes.* New York, NY: Henry Holt and Company, 1984. A self-care guide for the prevention and relief of athletic injuries.

Ornish, Dean, M.D. *Stress, Diet, and Your Heart.* New York, NY: Holt, Rinehart and Winston, 1982. Explores the connection between life-style and longevity.

Prevention Magazine Editors. *Understanding Vitamins and Minerals.* Emmons, PA: Rodale Press, 1983. A guide to nutritional needs.

Prudden, Bonnie. *Bonnie Prudden's Complete Guide to Pain-Free Living.* New York, NY: Ballantine Books, 1985. A self-help manual on pain control, emphasizing relaxation and muscular flexibility.

YOGA INSTRUCTION

To find a certified yoga teacher in your area, contact the Iyengar Yoga Institute, 2404 27th Avenue, San Francisco, California 94116. 415–753–0909.

BODYWORK TRAINING

Students interested in bodywork certification are urged to explore schools in Florida, New York, Arizona, and New Mexico. These states maintain commendable standards for schools and practitioners.

Before you enroll in any bodywork course, visit the school, speak with instructors, and take introductory classes. This will help you to determine whether the program will assist you in meeting your goals. Make sure that the required curriculum includes adequate amounts of anatomy, physiology, first aid, CPR certification, and other basic medical knowledge.

It is also helpful to determine the location in which you want to practice; familiarize yourself with its regulations concerning bodywork before planning your education.

References

1. TOUCH FOR HEALING: THE WESTERN VIEW OF ACUPRESSURE

Page 8   Dean Ornish, *Stress, Diet and Your Heart* (New York: Holt, Rinehart and Winston, 1982).

8   Richard Surwit and Michael Feinglos, "Relaxation-Induced Improvement in Glucose Tolerance is Associated with Decreased Plasma Cortisol," *Diabetes Care* (March–April 1984).

8   "Exclusive Interview with Henry Wingfield, Massage Therapist to Sugar Ray Leonard," *Massage* (Feb.–March 1988).

9   "Therapeutic Touch, the Imprimatur of Nursing," *Am. J. Nursing* 75 (1975): 784–87.

9   *Nursing Research* 30 (1985): 32–37.

9   David E. Bresler, et al., *Free Yourself from Pain* (New York: Simon and Schuster, Inc., 1979).

2. THE FIVE ELEMENTS: THE EASTERN VIEW OF ACUPRESSURE

Page 12   Bong-han study in Marc Duke, *Acupuncture* (New York: Harcourt Brace Jovanovich, 1972).

Page 13   *The Yellow Emperor's Classic of Internal Medicine,* Ilza Veith, trans. (Berkeley: University of California Press, 1966).

13   Peter Whybrow, et al., "The Hibernation Response," *New Age Journal* (Nov.–Dec. 1988).

4. COMMON AILMENTS A–Z

Page 41   *Medicine for Mountaineering,* James A. Wilkerson, ed. (Seattle, WA: The Mountaineers, 1985): 172–98.

44   Information on asthma in Brent Q. Hafen and Keith J. Karren, *Prehospital Emergency Care and Crisis Intervention* (Englewood, CO: Morton Publishing Co., 1983): 366–68.

45   Ben Benjamin, "The Mystery of Lower Back Pain," *Massage Therapy Journal* 27 (1988): 4.

48   Myles J. Schneider and Mark D. Sussman, *How to Doctor Your Feet without the Doctor* (New York: Charles Scribners' Sons, 1980), 91–94.

48   Information about boils in Joy Gardner, *The New Healing Yourself* (Freedom, CA: The Crossing Press, 1990), 45–46.

49   Information about bruises in Shizuko Yamamoto and Patrick McCarty, *Macrobiotic Family Health Care and Shiatsu* (Eureka, CA: Turning Point Publications), 91.

50   Information on burns from Wilkerson, 133–41.

52   I. Bonadeo and M. Lavazzo, "Echinacea B: polisacride attive dell'Echinacea," *Rev. Ital. Essenze Profumi* 53 (1981): 281–95.

55   "Cold Remedies: Which Ones Work Best?" *Consumer Reports* 54:1 (1989).

55   Information on cough suppressants: Ibid.

56   H. Wagner and A. Procksch, "An immunostimulating active principle from Echinacea Purpurea," *A. Agn. Physother.* 2:5 (1971): 166–78.

59   L. Lohmeier "The Hidden Addiction." *East West Journal* 18:3 (1988): 47.

Page 60   L. Cooper, "Constructive Living: Mastering the Morita Lifeway," *Yoga Journal* 80:16 (May–June 1988).

61   Fact sheet distributed by The Sjogren's Society, copyright © 1987.

78   Dr. Stan James in *The Physician and Sportsmedicine* 11:6 (1983): 201.

79   Robert Johnson quoted in J. Hogon, "The Most Common Ski Injury," *Snow Country*, (Dec. 1988): 32.

85   Dr. Richard A. Lannon in Charles Pettit, *San Francisco Chronicle* (Oct. 24 1987).

88   Information about poison in Hafen and Karren, 315–19.

90   S. B. Bittiner, et al., "A Double-Blind, Randomized Placebo-Controlled Trial of Fish Oil in Psoriasis," *Lancet* 1 (1988): 378–79.

92   Information on trauma in Hafen and Karren, 174.

94   On abdominal discomfort, see *The Biology of Alcoholism*, B. Kissin and H. Begleiter, eds. (New York: Plenum Publishing Co., 1974): 481–511; and F. B. Thomas, J. T. Steinbaugh, and J. J. Fromkes, et al., "Inhibitory Effect of Coffee on the Lower Esophageal Sphincter," *Gastroenterology* 79 (1980): 1262–66.

94   H. L. Green and F. K. Ghishan, "Excessive Fluid Intake as a Cause of Chronic Diarrhea in Young Children," *Journal of Pediatrics* 102 (1983): 836–39.

94   W. W. Feldman, P. McGrath, M. A. Hodgson, et al., "The Use of Dietary Fiber in the Management of Simple, Idiopathic Recurrent, Abdominal Pain: Results of a Prospective Double-Blind, Randomized, Controlled Trial," *American Journal of Digestive Disease* 139 (1985): 121–26.

95   H. Glatzel, "Treatment of Digestive Disorders with Spice Extracts," *Hippokrates* 40 (1969): 916–19.

95   E. H. Thompson, I. D. Wolk, and C. E. Allen, "Ginger Rhizome: a New Source of Proteolytic Enzyme," *Journal of Food Science* 38 (1973): 652–55.

109   H. Winter Griffith, *Complete Guide to Pediatric Symptoms, Illness, and Medication* (Los Angeles, CA: The Body Press, 1989), 356–357.

Index

Abdominal discomfort, 94–95
Abrasions, 40
Acidophilus, 84
Acne, 41
Affirmations, 44, 124, 128
Air pollution, 49, 61
Aloe vera gel, 40, 48, 51, 52, 62, 91, 106, 113, 124, 127
Alternatives in Medicine Clinic (Seattle), 59
Altitude sickness, 10, 41–42
American Association of Retired Persons (AARP), 120
Ampicillin, 55
Anal fissure, 42
Anaphylactic shock syndrome, 77
Anemia, iron-deficiency, 53, 66
Angina, 8, 25
Antibiotics, 55, 56, 62, 63, 83, 84, 117
Anxiety, 42–43
    breathing difficulties from, 49
    in hospitalized patients, 9

Arthritis, 3, 78
    rheumatoid, 61
Asthma, 44, 49
Ayurvedic medical practitioners, 8

Back pain and tension, 44–45
Balanitis, 45–46
Bed-wetting, see Urinary incontinence
Bee stings, see Insect stings
Benson, Herbert, 8
Biofeedback, 8
Blackheads, 41
Bladder meridian, 15, 47, 98
Bladder symptoms, 46–47
Bleeding, 47–48
Blisters, 48
Blood disorders, 17
Boils, 48–49
Boneset tea, 81
Bong-han, Kim, 12
Breastfeeding, 106
    boils and, 48

Breathing difficulties, 15, 44, 49
Bresler, David, 9
Brewer's yeast, 41
Bronchitis, 55–56
Bruises, 49–50
Bruxism, 50
Burns, 50–51
　blisters from, 47
Bursitis, *see* Joint pain and stiffness

Calcium, 50, 106
California, University of, at Los Angeles,
　Pain Control Unit at, 9
Calluses, 51–52
Calming meditation, 43, 44
Canker sores, 52
Carter, Jimmy and Rosalyn, 121
Chamomile, 56, 95
Chapped skin, 52
Chi, 12, 13
Chicken pox, 106–7
Children, 102–3
　chicken-pox in, 106–7
　convulsions in, 108–9
　croup in, 110
　fever in, 66–67
　hyperventilation in, 113–14
　impetigo in, 114
　measles in, 114–15
　mumps in, 115
　nosebleed in, 115–16
　shock in, 92
　stomach discomfort in, 94, 95
　tonsillitis in, 117
　vaginitis in, 118
Cholesterol, 8
Circulation problems, 16, 17, 53–54
Claustrophobia, 53
Clay masks, 127–28
Cold hands and feet, 53–54
Colds, 49, 54–55
Colic, 107
Comfrey, 76, 88

Concentration, lack of, 22
Conception Vessel, 17
Conjunctivitis, 56–57
Constipation, 57
　varicose veins and, 99
Constructive Living therapy, 60
Contact dermatitis, 58
Convulsions, 108–9
Corns, 51–52
Cornsilk tea, 47, 98
Coronary artery disease, 17
Corpse Revival, 65
Cradle cap, 109–10
Cramps, 58–59
　diarrhea and, 60
Croup, 110
Cystitis, 46

Dehydration, 100
　in infants, 111–12
Dental pain, 97
Depression, 25, 59–60
Dermatitis, contact, 58
Diabetes mellitus, 8
Diaper rash, 112–13
Diarrhea, 60–61
Diet
　depression and, 59, 60
　fatigue and, 66
　heat cramps and, 59
Digestive discomfort, 15
Disabled, 122–23
Disc problems, 45
Dolomite, 50
Dry eyes, 61
Duke University, 8
Dysentery, bacterial, 60

Ear discomfort, 61–62
Earth meridians, 14–15, 43, 46, 67, 85
Echinacea, 52, 67
Eczema, 62
Elimination problems, 15

Endorphins, 9, 60
Elderly, 119–23
    frail, 122–23
    self-treatment for, 120–21
    shock in, 92
Epididymitis, 63
Excessive perspiration, 63–64
Exercise, 124
    circulation and, 53
    constipation and, 57
    depression relieved by, 60
    foot pain and, 68
    heat loss during, 58, 59
    joint pain and, 78
    stitch in side during, 93–94
    varicose veins and, 99
Eyes
    dry, 61
    exercises to strengthen, 64
    foreign object in, 65
    infection of, 56–57
Eyestrain, 64

Facial tension, 41
Fainting, 65
Fatigue, 65–66
    during labor, 9
    post-surgical, 3
Feet
    cold, 53–54
    pain in, 68
Fennel, 126
Fever, 66–67
    convulsions and, 108
Fight or flight syndrome, 8
Fire meridians, 16–17, 46, 54, 67, 75,
    99
Fish oil, 91
Five Elements Theory, 2, 3, 12–17
Flatulence, 67–68
Flu, 75–76
Food poisoning, 60
Foreskin inflammation, 45–46

Gall Bladder meridian, 16
Gastric ulcers, 8
Gastroenteritis, 21
Gatorade, 111
Genital herpes, 73
Gingerroot, 46, 54, 63, 90, 95
Glycerine soap, 42, 48
Goldenseal, 57, 58, 73, 74
Golden Points, 19, 26, 28, 31–32
Gout, 69
Governing Vessel, 17
Green-clay paste, 49, 52, 73, 90
Grey Panthers, 120
Grief, 15
Gynecological treatment, 4

Habitat for Humanity, 121
Hands, cold, 53–54
Harvard University, 8
Hayes, Helen, 96
Hay fever, 69–70
Headache, 70–71
    migraine, 2, 8, 99
Healing Arts, The (Kaptchuk), 13
Heartburn, 71
Heart meridian, 16
Heat cramps, 58
Heel spurs, 68
Hemorrhoids, 71
Herbalism, 3, 10, 124–27
    for colds, 55–56
Hernia, 72–73
Herpes, 73
Hiatal hernia, 72
Hives, 73–74
Holistic healing, 2, 125
    for depression, 59
Hot flashes, 121–22
Hypertension, 17
    stress and, 8
Hyperventilation, 113–14
Hypnosis, 8
Hypoglycemia, 66

Ice, 128
Impetigo, 114
Impotence, 74–75
Incisional hernia, 72
Infants, 102–3
    breastfeeding, 106
    colic in, 107
    cradle cap in, 109–10
    dehydration in, 111–12
    diaper rash in, 112–13
    teething in, 116–17
    touch-sensitive, 111
    umbilical cord infection in, 117–18
Influenza, 75–76
    vertigo in, 99
Inguinal hernia, 72
Injection pain, 76
Insect stings, 1, 76–77
Insensitivity, 17
Insomnia, 77
    in children, 102
Iron-deficiency anemia, 53, 66
Isolation, 17
Iyengar yoga, 78

James, Stan, 78
Jock rot, 77–78
Johnson, Robert, 79
Joint pain and stiffness, 78–79
Jojoba oil, 52, 91

Kaptchuk, Ted, 13
Kidney meridian, 15, 47, 98
Knee injury, 79–80
Krieger, Dolores, 19

Langley-Porter Neuropsychiatric Institute, 85
Lannon, Richard A., 85
Large Intestine meridian, 15, 41
Laryngitis, 81–82
Leonard, Sugar Ray, 8–9
Licorice root, 111

Liver meridian, 16, 52
Liver pain, 82
Lung meridian, 15

Macrobiotics, 69
Magnesium, 50
Marigold poultice, 48
Massage, 8–11, 91–92
Measles, 114–15
Medical emergencies
    breathing difficulties in, 49
    in children, 108, 109
    shock as, 92
Meditation, 86
    calming, 43, 44
    walking, 81
Menopausal symptoms, 4, 121–22
Menstrual discomfort, 3, 4
    cramps, 58–59, 83
Mental imaging, 8, 124, 130
Meridians, 12–17
Metal meridians, 15, 67, 91, 107, 112
Migraine headache, 2
    stress and, 8
    vertigo and, 99
Mint tea, 61, 67, 81, 85, 100
Monilia, 83–84
    antibiotics and, 52
Montezuma's Revenge, 60
Morita, Shoma, 60
Morning sickness, 95
Mugwort, 82
Mumps, 115

Nasal congestion, 84
Natural products, 127–28
Nausea, 84–85
Neural receptors, 9–10
Neuroma, 3
New York City Ballet, 66
Nichols, Kyra, 66
Nosebleed, 115–16
Nurse-midwives, 9

Ornish, Dean, 8

Pain relief, 2, 11
   in arthritis, 3
   in chronic conditions, 3–4
   during labor, 9
Panic, 85–86
Pelvic pain, 86–87
Pennsylvania, University of, 13
Pericardium meridian, 16
Perspiration, excessive, 63–64
Pharyngitis, 87–88
Phelps, Janice, 59–60
Pimples, 41
Pinkeye, 56–57
Poison exposure or ingestion, 88–89
Poison oak, ivy, or sumac, 89–90
Pomeranz, Bruce, 9
Post-surgical fatigue, 3
Potato suppository, 71
Pregnancy
   acupressure points to avoid during, 18, 20, 23, 24
   heartburn during, 71
   hemorrhoids during, 71
   herbs to avoid during, 58, 74
   morning sickness during, 95
   rubella during, 114–15
   shock during, 92
   stitch in side during, 93
   varicose veins during, 98
Premenstrual syndrome, 4, 15
   acne and, 41
   back pain in, 45
Prickly heat, 112–13
Prostate symptoms, 90
Psoriasis, 90–91
Psychiatric care, 59
Pyoderma, 114

Rape, 87
Rash, 58
Recurrent Abdominal Pain (RAP), 94

Reflexology, 123
Relation techniques, 7, 8
Reye's syndrome, 106–7, 109, 115, 117
Rheumatoid arthritis, 61
RICE technique, 79–80, 91
Rose clay mask, 41

Scrapes, 40
Scrotum inflammation and infection, 63
Seasonal Affective Disorder (SAD), 13
Self-esteem, low, 17, 59, 60
Self-care instruction, 5
   for elderly, 120–21
Selye, Hans, 7–8
Sexual dysfunction, 23
Shiatsu, 2, 3, 8, 10–11
Shingles, 107
Shin splints, 91–92
Shock, 19, 92–93
Sjogren's Syndrome, 61
Skin
   chapped, 52
   dry, 91
Sleeplessness, 77
Small Intestine meridian, 16, 52
Smoke inhalation, 93
Sore throat, 87–88
Spinal discomfort, 44–45
Spleen meridian, 14, 43
Sports injury, prevention of, 80
Stitch in side, 94
Stomach discomfort, 94–95
Stomach meridian, 14, 43
Strep throat, 88
Stress, Diet and Your Heart (Ornish), 8
Stress reduction, 3, 7–8, 95–96
   for hives, 74
   for panic attacks, 85–86
Stretching, 45, 54, 124, 128, 129
Surgery, 11
   fatigue following, 3
Swedish/Esalen massage, 2

Tai Chi Chu'an, 3
Taoism, 13
Teething, 116–17
Temporomandibular Joint Syndrome, 50, 70
Tendonitis, 96
Tennis elbow, 96
Tension relief, 2, 11
  back, 44–45
  facial, 41
  during labor, 9
Testicle torsion, 97
Therapeutic Touch, 9
Three burning spaces, 16
Three More Miles, 66
Tonsillitis, 117
Toothache, 97
Tooth grinding, 50
Toronto, University of, 9
Touch therapies, 2, 9, 10
  for children, 103
Trichomonas, 83
Triple Warmer meridian, 16

Umbilical cord infection, 117–18
Umbilical hernia, 72

Urinary disorders, 66
Urinary incontinence, 98
  insomnia and, 77

Vaginismus, 86
Vaginitis, 83
  in children, 118
Valerian root, 125
Varicose veins, 98–99
Venereal disease, bladder symptoms in, 47
Vermont, University of, 79
Vertigo, 99
Visualization, 3, 124, 128, 130
Volunteer work, 121
Vomiting, 100

Water meridians, 15, 46, 62, 75, 99
Walking meditation, 81
Wheelchair users, 122
Whiplash, 100–101
Wood meridians, 16, 61
Wounds, bleeding, 47

Yeast infections, *see* Monilia
Yin and yang, 13–16
Yoga, 78, 124